d·i·y Updos, Knots, & Twists

Easy, Step-by-Step Styling Instructions
for 35 Hairstyles
from Inverted Fishtails to Polished Ponytails!

MELISSA COOK *of www.missysue.com*

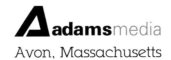

Aadamsmedia
Avon, Massachusetts

DEDICATION

To my family, who supports me in all my endeavors and
reminds me I can do anything I set my mind to. I love you!

Published by
Adams Media, a division of F+W Media, Inc.
57 Littlefield Street, Avon, MA 02322. U.S.A.
www.adamsmedia.com

ISBN 10: 1-4405-8875-9
ISBN 13: 978-1-4405-8875-4
eISBN 10: 1-4405-8876-7
eISBN 13: 978-1-4405-8876-1

Printed in the United States of America.

10   9   8   7   6   5   4   3   2   1

Library of Congress Cataloging-in-Publication Data

Cook, Melissa.
  DIY updos, knots, & twists / Melissa Cook of *www.missysue.com*.
    pages cm
  Includes index.
  ISBN 978-1-4405-8875-4 (pob) -- ISBN 1-4405-8875-9 (pob) -- ISBN 978-1-4405-8876-1 (ebook) -- ISBN
1-4405-8876-7 (ebook)
  1. Braids (Hairdressing) 2. Long hair styling. I. Title. II. Title: Do it yourself updos, knots, and twists.
  TT975.C657 2015
  646.7'247--dc23

                            2015019040

Cover design by Stephanie Hannus.
Photos by Melissa Cook.

This book is available at quantity discounts for bulk purchases.
For information, please call 1-800-289-0963.

Contents

Introduction

Are you stuck in a rut with that boring pony-tail and basic bun? Not sure how to amp up your style? Do you think braids, updos, and twists are just too difficult to incorporate into your everyday look?

If this sounds like you, the styles found in *DIY Updos, Knots, & Twists* are going to change your look for the better! Here you will find more than thirty hairstyles ranging from twisted looks, like the Twists to Bun in Chapter 2; to intricate buns like the Double-Wrapped Bun in Chapter 3; to embellished braids, like the Inverted Fishtail Updo in Chapter 4; to upscale ponys like the Twisted Low Ponytail in Chapter 5. In addition, you'll find a chapter that teaches you everything you need to know to successfully create the various updos in this book, including information on the materials you should have on hand as well as various techniques like how to reduce flyaways, back-comb your hair to add volume, get the perfect curl, and more!

So how can you master these on-trend, beautiful hairstyles? That's actually the number one question I'm asked all the time! Was I born with the talent? Is my hair different somehow? The truth is that all it takes is prac-tice, practice, practice. The more you practice these styles on your medium to long hair and wear these hairstyles out and about, the more confident you will feel doing them. Read each step carefully, follow along as I show you how to make these fun and chic styles, check your work in the mirror as you go, and soon peo-ple will be amazed by your skills! You will feel more confident in your ability because you will know you look great. Whether you have fine, thick, curly, or straight hair, pretty soon you will be able to create such beautiful, intri-cate styles that all the looks in this book will be easy-peasy and you can start to show your friends how to create them too.

My hope is that this book will inspire you to really get to know your hair, to play around with it more often and discover and try out new ways to wear it. I hope it will help you improve your skills at creating these styles—but most of all, I hope this book will encour-age you to be confident in your ability to do your hair, and to love and enjoy it as I have learned to love my own.

CHAPTER 1

Tips and Tricks for the Perfect Updo

Creating that perfect updo takes practice but knowing the right tips and tricks can make it ten times easier to accomplish. The techniques explained in this chapter will help you achieve beautiful styles, whether it is with the right amount of back-combing, the perfect texture of curls, or knowing when to use an elastic band versus a bobby pin. Learning if a comb or brush is more helpful in creating a smooth style and which hairspray is the right one to reach for will be useful in creating a finished look that will make you feel confident in your hairstyling abilities.

Materials You Will Need

Here you'll find information on the basic tools and hair appliances you'll need in your beauty arsenal. They include the necessary items for completing each style in the book as well as a few useful pieces to help you give each style a polished and perfected finish.

» **Wide-tooth comb:** for untangling and straightening wet or dry hair. This type of comb has teeth that are well spaced apart and is great for all hair textures and lengths.

» **Paddle brush:** wide, flat brush with soft bristles. This type of brush is best for medium to long hair to help smooth it down and tame flyaways. It works well on curly, frizzy, or wavy hair and is great for penetrating thick hair while providing a gentle scalp massage.

» **Teasing brush:** used to back-comb the hair. Learn more about back-combing in the "Techniques" section later in this chapter.

» **Hairbands (also called hair ties):** fabric-covered bands, 2" in diameter, used to secure large sections of hair. This type of band can be used on any hair type but works especially well with

thick, coarse, or curly hair. These can be purchased at your local grocery store or beauty supply store. The metal-free type work best to ensure the least amount of hair breakage or damage.

» **Clear elastic bands:** reusable, plastic, stretchy bands, ½–1" in diameter, used to secure small sections of hair. This type of band is best used to tie off the end of a braid or twist, to separate small sections of hair, or when a portion of a hairstyle needs to be hidden or less noticeable, such as with a topsy tail. These can be purchased in the hair aisle of your local grocery store or beauty supply store.

» **Bobby pins, also known as hair grips:** small pieces of metal bent into two prongs pressed close together, about 2" in length. These pins are used by slightly opening the prongs and sliding them over small sections of hair, with the bumpy side against the head, and then the prongs close over the hair, holding it in place.

» **Hair donut:** stretchy, easy-to-use donut-shaped bun holder that adds fullness and shape to updos. This can be used for all hair types and be purchased to match your hair color.

» **Stretchy headband:** fabric-covered, circular headband used to hold the hair back from the face, generally 6–7" in diameter.

» **Duck-bill clip:** lightweight metal clip with coil springs, about 3–4" in length, used to secure hair after it is sectioned off.

» **Flexible-hold hairspray:** maintains style with a soft, natural finish. This type of hairspray is ideal for holding curls while still allowing for movement. It helps keep hair under control without stiffness and is perfect for everyday use. To effectively hold the hair in place, spray a mist of hairspray all around the head for 3–4 seconds.

» **Medium-hold hairspray:** provides a stronger hold than flexible-hold hairspray, but allows movement with minimal stiffness when applied sparingly. This type is ideal for soft, looser updos and for half updos where sections of hair are pinned up and the rest is left down.

» **Maximum-hold hairspray:** the strongest of all the hairsprays and ideal for dramatic updos. It helps keep every strand in place for hours at a time.

The items on this list are all essentials that every woman needs in her beauty kit. They will help you create smooth, refined styles for every day of the week.

Extra Items to Consider

Mastering that perfect hairstyle always takes a bit of practice, and the items on this list can help make achieving it a little bit easier. They are not necessary or required for everyday use but can be helpful to have on hand. These are all best used in moderation and should be applied a little bit at a time—think pea-size to nickel-size amounts. Of course, more can always be added if needed. Remember that it's easier to add more product than it is to remove the excess after it has been applied.

» **Spray wax:** non-oily spray that creates bendable textures. This product is ideal for laying flat the short, broken hairs that tend to stick up, especially along the part. It delivers a satin finish, but applying too much can weigh down the hair and make it heavy. To apply this product, hold the bottle at least 12" from the head and use in moderation.

- » **Pomade:** waxy substance used to make hair look slick and shiny, and reduce frizz. This product is ideal for making short hairstyles stay upright. For application on updos, use a pea-size amount and gently massage it between the thumb and pointer finger before smoothing it over random hairs that stick out from a style, to slick them down and keep them in place.

- » **Shine serum:** substance applied to the ends of damp hair before styling to protect against dryness, smooth down frizz, and give the appearance of shiny, moisturized hair.

- » **Hair oil:** lightweight oil used to deeply hydrate and treat hair. Use hair oil as a leave-in conditioner by applying it to damp or dry hair from the mid-shaft down. Brush through the hair to evenly distribute the oil through the hair. Avoid the scalp area; used there, it can make hair greasy and weigh it down. A nickel-size amount is ideal for long hair and less for shorter hair.

- » **Dry shampoo:** a dry substance that works by absorbing oil from the scalp and making it look freshly washed in order to lengthen the time between washes. It comes in three forms: powder, liquid in a pump dispenser, or aerosol spray.

- » **Heat serum:** non-oily spray used to protect hair from heat damage caused by curling irons, straighteners, and blow dryers. On wet hair, spray the hair from the roots to the ends before blow-drying. Once the hair is dry, mist it all again before heat styling to reduce the damage caused by hot tools.

- » **1" curling iron:** creates a tight, defined curl, rather than loose waves. This curl is perfect for short to medium-length hair.

- » **1½" curling iron:** creates a loose, casual curl.

- » **Straightener:** heats up hair to straighten kinks, waves, and curls. It is also used to reduce frizz and create shiny straight hair.

With these extra items and a little practice, you will have all the tools needed to perfect each style in this book.

Techniques

In this section, you'll learn a few of the basic methods for making each style look more professional and polished. These techniques are referenced throughout the book in the styles that use them; you can return to this section for the detailed explanation of the techniques as needed.

Back-Comb or "Tease" Hair

To add volume to any style, you want to first tease or back-comb the hair:

1. Separate off a 1" horizontal section of hair at the middle of the crown. Lift the hair upwards so it points straight up from the scalp, place a teasing brush horizontally at the midpoint of the section, and gently push the hair downwards towards the scalp. Repeat this 3–4 times or until the majority of the hair is brushed downwards.

2. Next, spray the underside of the section near the root, so it's evenly coated with a medium-hold hairspray, for about 1 second, and position it upside down so the ends lie towards the face or over the forehead. Leave it there while you work on a new section and becomes dry to the touch.

3. Repeat the previous step with 2–3 more sections of hair or until you reach the back of the crown, so all the hair at the crown of the head is teased.

4. Gently lift up the teased sections and direct them towards the back of the head. Carefully comb through the topmost layer of hair so the portion that is teased is hidden underneath smoothed hair.

Curl Your Hair

Curling your hair before starting to style it will make creating any updo easier! It helps because the hair can be styled uniformly rather than as a mix of random textures, such as straight sections mixed with wavy sections if your hair doesn't naturally dry evenly. The following steps work for any size curling iron and any hair texture. Of course, if you have naturally curly hair and it is all the same texture, then you can skip this section. For everyday curls and to prep for any style in this book:

1. Start by spraying all the hair with a heat serum and combing through it to evenly distribute the product.

2. Divide the hair into three sections; one from the temples to the back of the crown and one from the top of each ear to the back of the head, clipping off the top two sections.

3. With your dominant hand on the handle of the iron, use your other hand to pick up a 1" section of unclipped hair from behind one ear. Open the clamp with your pointer finger and close it on the middle of the section of hair, holding the curling iron vertical with the tip pointing upwards and the clamp facing forwards.

4. Twist the curling iron towards the back of the head, away from the face, wrapping the hair around the barrel as you twist until it's about 1" from the scalp.

5. Gently feel the hair wrapped around the barrel until it is hot to the touch. You can also count to 5 if you have fine, thin hair; 8 if you have fine, thick hair; or 10 if you have course, thick hair.

6. Using your pointer finger, gently loosen the clamp and slide the iron down to the bottom of the section of hair.

7. Release the clamp on the end of the hair and repeat Steps 3–6, rolling the curling iron vertically, towards the back of the head, until it reaches the halfway point. Curling your hair in halves this way will ensure that each section is evenly curled and reduce the amount of damage caused by the heat.

8. Repeat these steps with the remaining hair, letting down the next pinned section and curling it the same way.

9. Finish by curling the topmost section of hair.

10. Apply hair oil to the ends of the hair to add moisture and reduce heat damage caused by the hot tool.

Add Volume to Braids

If you have fine or thin hair and want to make your braids appear thicker, this is a quick trick to achieve just that. This is also a very modern way to style a braid, giving the appearance of a very voluminous and editorial style. This method of volumizing a braid is always optional and not required for completing any of these styles.

1. Divide off a 2" section of hair on the heavy side of the part. Create a basic braid, by separating the section into three equal sections. Cross the left section over the middle so the middle piece now becomes the left-sided piece and the left piece now becomes the middle; essentially they switch places. Now cross the strand on the right side over the middle, so the middle and right switch places. Repeat the previous steps, crossing the left over the middle then the right over the middle until reaching the end of the section.

2. Tie off the end with a clear elastic band.

3. Holding on to the elastic band with one hand, gently pull up one side of the braid so the hair slowly comes loose from the elastic and doubles in size, or until the piece looks wide and flat. Switch hands and loosen the other side.

4. Carefully work your way up the braid, pulling the edges looser so they are wider and flatter.

5. Slide the hairband up the braid or pull it off and then replace it on the hair so the new, wider braid maintains its shape. It is always best to loosen a little at a time, working up to the top, and then start over again at the bottom, pulling it looser still. If you pull the braid too wide and it falls apart, simply re-braid the section and begin again.

Reduce Stray Hairs and Smooth Flyaways

With many hairstyles and updos, there are always a few stray hairs that stick out of the top of the head or somehow work their way out of a wrapped style and hang loose. There are also small, shorter hairs that stick up around the hairline and along the part. This is most apparent in hair that is color-treated and has experienced a lot of breakage, but it is also seen with hair that experiences a lot of heat styling, which causes damage and breakage. For people with curly hair, this may always be an issue because the strands often do not lie smoothly or uniformly together. There are a few tricks you can do to hide any small hairs that stick up from a hairstyle. These steps are not necessarily required, but they're great if you want to achieve a polished finish.

1. Comb through the hair with a wide-tooth comb to remove any tangles.

2. Spray the top and sides of the head with a medium-hold hairspray. Be sure to hold it about 12" away from the head.

3. Immediately (while it is still wet) comb through the hair again with the wide-tooth comb.

4. Continue combing the hair, then sweep it into a ponytail or bun.

5. After finishing any style, spray your fingertips with hairspray and glide them over any stray hairs that stick out of the style.

Add Texture to Fine Hair

Fine hair means that individual hairs are very skinny. It is possible to have thin, fine hair or thick, fine hair. Either way, this type of hair is the most prone to tangles and is slippery in texture, and therefore difficult to keep in place. The techniques given here will solve this issue, helping thin hair hold any style.

1. Spray a small amount of dry shampoo along the part, then create a second part next to it, flipping the hair over to the opposite side of the head, and spray the roots again. Continue sectioning the hair this way until reaching the ear. Then return the hair back to its natural direction and repeat the previous steps with the hair on the other side of the part. Let the hair dry for a few minutes, then comb through it with a wide-tooth comb to help distribute the product throughout the hair. This will help create a bit of texture and grip.

2. Back-comb or tease the hair before beginning any style.

3. Use a flexible- or medium-hold hairspray and steer clear of heavy gels or wax

sprays, which can greatly weigh down your fine tresses.

4. Before beginning any style, curl your hair, referring to the instructions in the "Curl Your Hair" technique, which can help the hair appear thicker and fuller than it is.

Make Curly or Coarse Hair Easy to Style

Curly or coarse hair can be difficult to work with because usually there is a lot of it and it doesn't want to do what you would like it to. Curly hair can stick out in odd places and be difficult to tame. Coarse hair can be hard to curl or very heavy, making it difficult to maintain its shape. Here are a few tips and tricks to make hair that seems unmanageable easier to work with:

1. Work with hair a day or two after washing it. Natural oils help styles stay in better than they do in freshly washed hair, which can be slippery.

2. Apply heavier products such as gels, pomades, or shine serum to cut down on frizz and help the style stay and hold better.

3. Use more bobby pins than what is recommended. Curly, thick hair is heavy,

and adding a few extra pins will ensure that the style stays all day.

4. When braiding, twisting, and pinning any section of hair, pull it a little extra tight. Your fullness will naturally create a bigger style, and it's easier to loosen a style once it's done than to try to tighten it back up.

5. Have your stylist cut long layers at your next haircut. This will give the hair movement and help thin it out a little. Do some research about what you want beforehand, though, and make sure the layers don't start any higher than your cheekbones.

Now that you know what you will need to have on hand, and have learned a few tricks for solving issues that may come your way, you're ready to try out the thirty-five updos, knots, and twists found in the following chapters. If at any time you run into a problem or have a question, you can come back to this chapter, read up on these tools and tips, and give it another go. Good luck, have fun, and enjoy your new updos!

CHAPTER 2

High Buns and Mid Buns

High buns and mid buns are perfect for every day because they can be dressed up for a date or worn casually for work or a lunch with friends. To achieve these styles, it is important to have mastered the technique behind a high ponytail, where combing all the hair upwards towards the crown and securing it in place is required, as well as a regular ponytail that aligns with the ears. A comb or brush is always required for these styles, because smoothing the hair around the head is how a sleek style will be achieved each time. Doing this in combination with using hairspray to flatten out any hair that sticks up will ensure a sophisticated-looking updo each time.

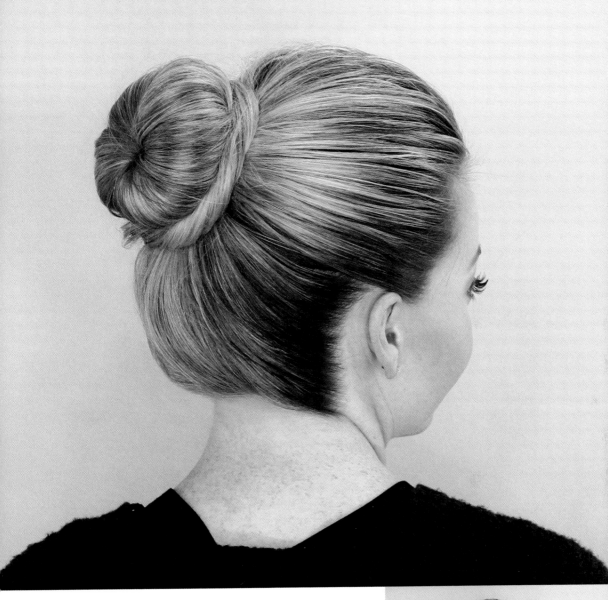

Donut Bun

This bun is probably the easiest one you will ever do. Why? Because a hair donut underneath the hair creates the perfect guide for making a simple, sleek hairstyle. And once you get this technique down, you'll realize how easy it is to create fun variations by wrapping the bun with a braid or adding an extra detail such as a hair accessory. Grab your hairspray and give it a try!

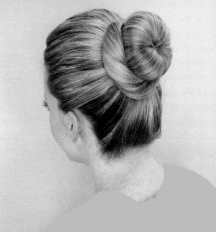

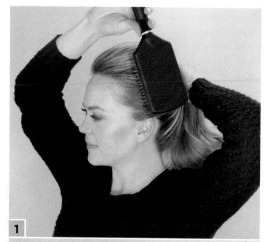

1

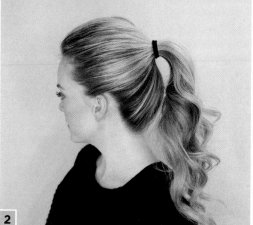

2

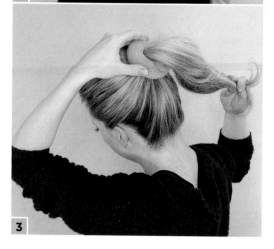

3

MATERIALS

» Paddle brush
» Medium-hold hairspray
» 1 hairband
» Hair donut
» 1 clear elastic band
» 1–4 bobby pins

1. Use a paddle brush to smooth all the hair back into a high ponytail. For a smooth look, spray the hair with hairspray before brushing it.

2. Tie off the hair using a hairband. Make sure the ponytail sits high on the head, at the back of the crown, above the ears.

3. Slide a hair donut over the ponytail so it sits over the hairband.

4. Angle the head downwards, with the chin towards the chest so the donut is resting on top of the head. Spread out the pony-tail and cover the hair donut evenly with it, securing it with your hand at the base of the bun. The hair should be completely covering the hair donut so it is hidden underneath it. Slide a clear elastic band over the top to keep the hair in place. Spray the bun with hairspray and slide your hands over the shape of the bun to smooth down any stray hairs.

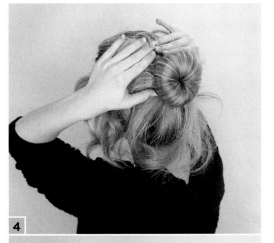

5. Combine all the hair that is hanging out from the bun and twist it together.

6. Wrap the twist around the base of the bun and pin the end to hold it in place. Slide the pin into the bun to hide it. Then spray the style with hairspray to set it while smoothing down any loose hairs.

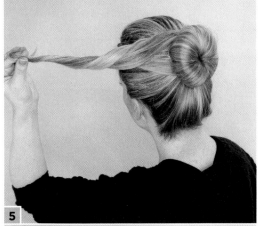

UPDO EXTRAS

When twisting the extra hair hanging out from the bun, roll it into a tight twist before wrapping it. It is easier to make it larger afterwards than smaller after pinning.

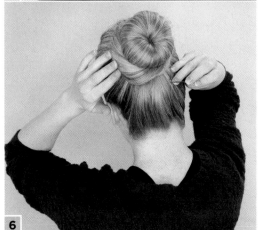

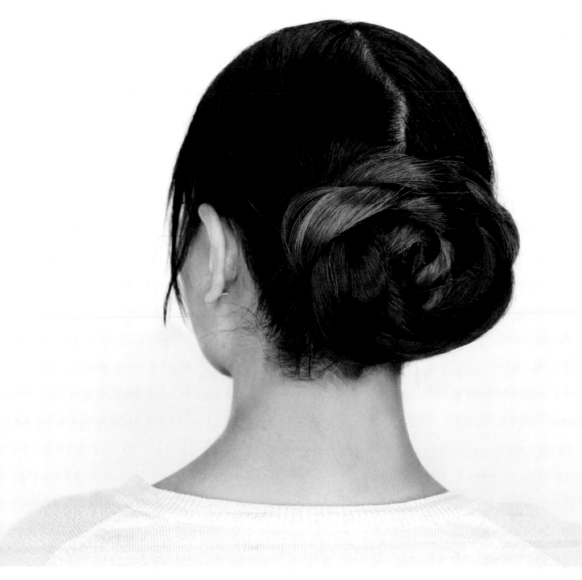

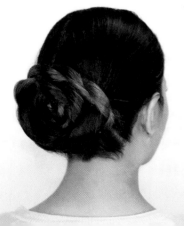

Twisted Bun

A new take on the everyday chignon, this hairstyle is a great way to dress up your everyday bun. It's created by twisting two ponytails into rope braids that are then twisted around each other to make this intricate-looking bun. This Twisted Bun is a gorgeous style that is perfect for the office or a night out with friends, so feel free to dress it up with heels or down with casual jeans. Either way, you're guaranteed to look amazing!

MATERIALS

» Wide-tooth comb
» 4 clear elastics bands
» 6–8 bobby pins
» Maximum-hold hairspray

1. Begin by creating a part down the center of the back of the head, dividing the hair into two halves, left and right. Tie off each side with a clear elastic band to create two ponytails at the back of the head, lining them up with the top of the ears.

2. Take one ponytail and separate it into two strands. Twist each strand away from the face, then wrap the strands around each other in the opposite direction, creating a rope braid. Tie off the end with a clear elastic band.

3. Repeat the previous step with the second ponytail, creating another rope braid and tying off the end with an elastic band.

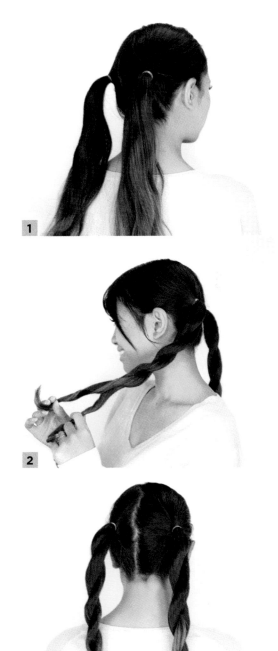

4. Take the left rope braid and wrap it into a bun so it sits at the center of the back of the head, between the two braids. Pin it in place with bobby pins.

5. Take the other rope and wrap it around the outside of the first bun.

6. Secure the entire bun by sliding pins over the various sections, towards the center. Then set the style with hairspray and smooth down any stray hairs.

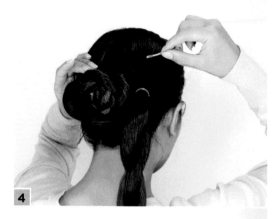

UPDO EXTRAS

After creating the ponytails, spray them with hairspray and run a comb through the hair to smooth down any flyaways. To ensure that the finished style is sleek, wrap the hair tightly when creating the rope braids, then spray the braid with hairspray and smooth down any flyaways after tying off the end with the elastic.

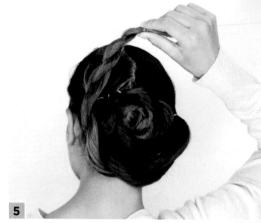

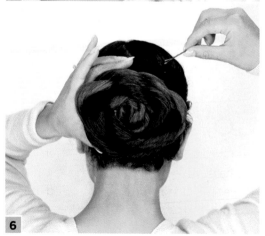

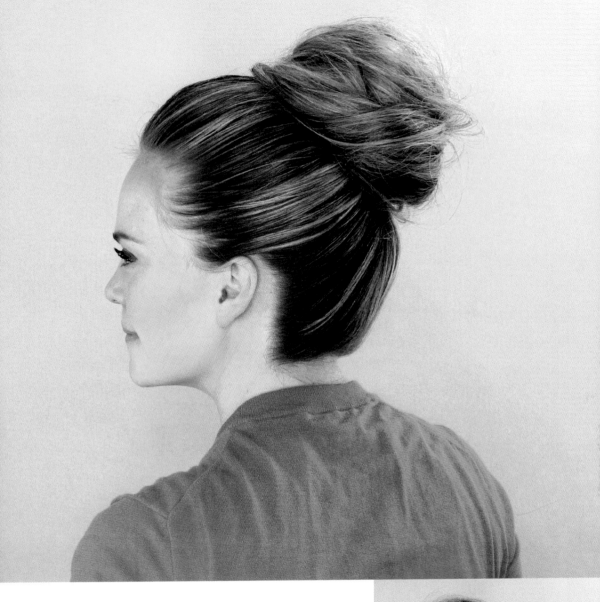

Cotton Candy Bun

The Cotton Candy Bun is a modern version of the topknot. This hairstyle is a staple and is one that you will come back to over and over again. In this on-trend hairstyle, the effect of cotton candy is created by back-combing all the hair in the ponytail, then gently smoothing it into a wrapped bun. It only takes seconds to do and can be worn pretty much anywhere. Enjoy!

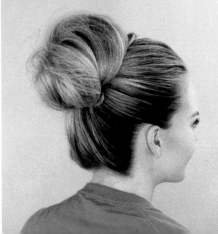

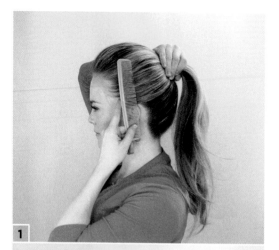

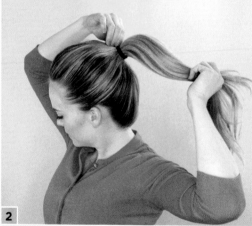

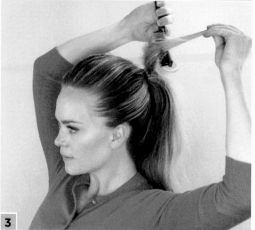

MATERIALS

» Wide-tooth comb
» Maximum-hold hairspray
» 1 hairband
» Teasing brush
» 2–5 bobby pins

1. Start by combing the hair back into a high ponytail. For a sleeker effect, comb the hair back and spray the top and sides with hairspray before combing over it again. This will smooth down flyaways and create a more seamless look.

2. Tie off the hair with a hairband.

3. Next, grab a teasing brush and gently back-comb the ponytail in small sections; 3–4 sections for thinner hair and 5–6 sections for thicker hair. The trick to a gentle back-comb is to push the hair down towards the hairband. Start the comb at the middle of the strand and push the hair downwards before sliding the brush straight back up and repeating the downward strokes until the entire strand is teased.

4. Continue back-combing until all the strands are combed. Remember that the goal is to create volume, so the bigger the tease the better. Then take the entire ponytail and give it a quick spray with hairspray before twisting it forwards.

5. Wrap the hair around the hairband, forming a bun. Slide pins around the base of the bun to secure the hair. Sliding the pins towards the elastic band will ensure they remain out of view at the end. Then set the finished style with a liberal spray of hairspray, smoothing down the hair leading to the bun and the bun itself.

UPDO EXTRAS

Start out by making the bun smaller than you'd like because it can always be pulled looser at the end. If it doesn't work exactly right the first time, remove the pins and twist it again. Sometimes it can take a few tries before the preferred shape is achieved.

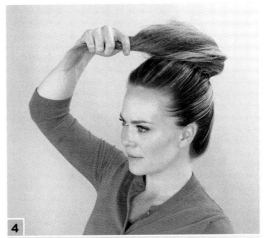

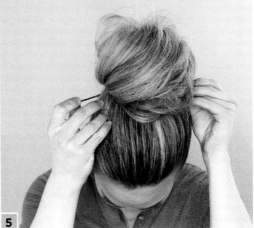

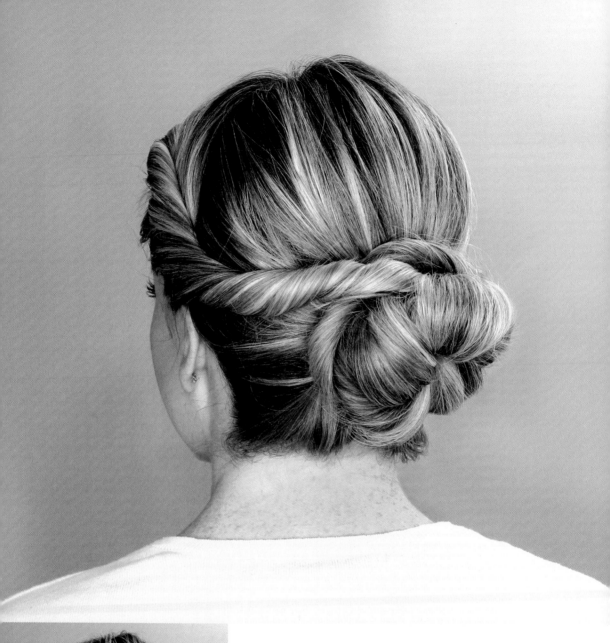

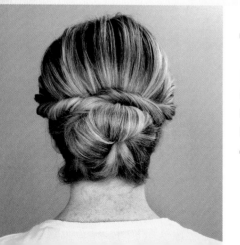

Twists to Bun

If you are looking for a great way to jazz up your bun but braiding isn't your thing, then this Twists to Bun style will become your new favorite mid bun updo. Create this style by sectioning and twisting your hair into a chic bun. It's quick, easy, and perfect for every day of the week.

MATERIALS

» Wide-tooth comb
» 2 duck-bill clips
» 8–10 bobby pins
» Maximum-hold hairspray

1. Start by separating the hair into three sections. Create a part from the top of the crown down to the ear, clipping off the front portion with a duck-bill clip. Now create a second part on the opposite side, clipping off the front portion again with another clip.

2. Pick up the back section of hair and twist all the hair in that section into a sleek bun at the center of the back of the head, so it lines up with the top of the ears.

3. Secure the bun with bobby pins by sliding them towards the center of the bun and hiding them underneath. Use as many pins as you need; I like to use at least six pins. You may need less than that if your hair is thin, or more if your hair is very thick.

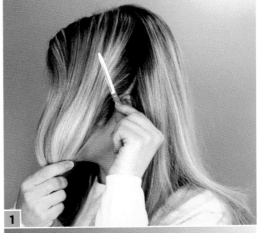

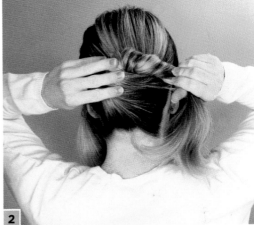

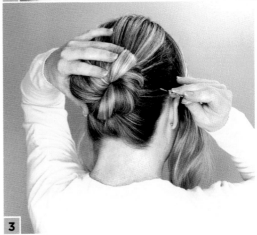

4. Remove the clip holding the right front portion of hair and twist the hair upwards towards the back of the head. Add in hair as you work your way towards the back of the head until all the hair is brought in.

5. Lay the twist over the top of the bun and wrap it counter-clockwise around the bun.

6. Secure the tail of the twist by pinning it underneath the bun, sliding the pin towards the middle of the bun.

7. Now create a second twist with the hair on the left side of the head. Lay it over the bun as before and wrap it clockwise around the bun.

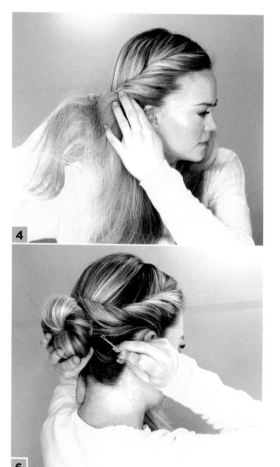

4

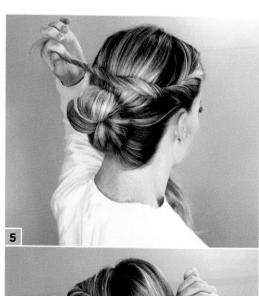

5

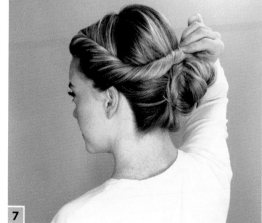

6

7

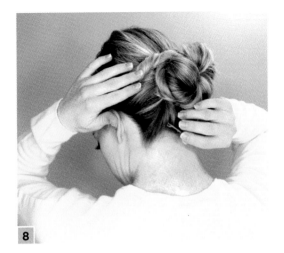

8. Pin down the end of the twist, hiding it underneath the bun, then set the style with hairspray and smooth down any stray hairs.

UPDO EXTRAS

To create a smooth bun and twists, spray the hair first with hairspray and comb through it to remove any tangles. When rolling the hair for the bun and twists, keep it tight so it doesn't come loose. It is easier to loosen them up afterwards than to make them tighter.

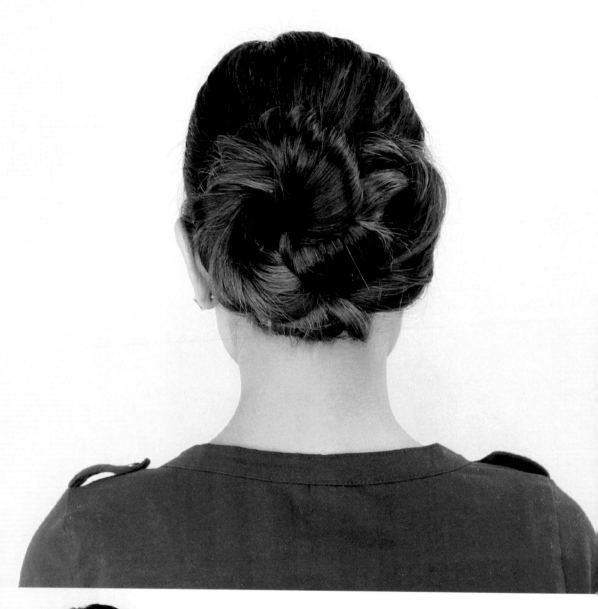

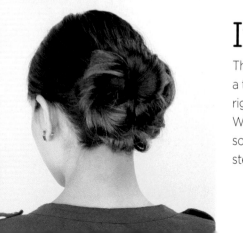

Infinity Bun

This Infinity Bun is a little tricky to master, because it requires a tight grip on the hair and a bit of maneuvering to get the right shape. With a bit of practice though it can be done. When creating this updo, work with the ponytail in sections so the twist is easier to work with. Once you've mastered the steps, you will love the unique shape and design of the bun.

MATERIALS

» Paddle brush
» Maximum-hold hairspray
» 1 clear elastic band
» Wide-tooth comb
» 8–10 bobby pins

1. Start by brushing the hair back into a ponytail that lines up with the top of the ears. For a sleek look, brush the hair back and spray the top and sides with hairspray before brushing over it again. This smooths down flyaways and creates a more seamless look. Tie off the hair with a clear elastic band. Then comb through the ponytail to remove any tangles.

2. Divide the ponytail into two halves, a top and a bottom. Twist the top portion upwards for the first part of the infinity.

3. Next, lay the twist against the head to make the first part of the infinity symbol. It should create a "C" type shape. Pin down the twist with bobby pins as you go so it maintains its shape.

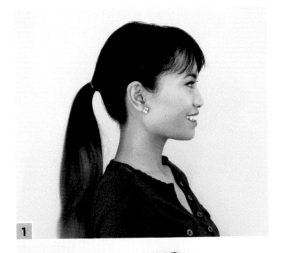

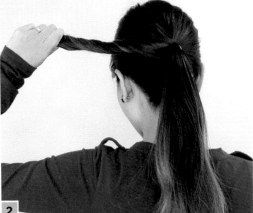

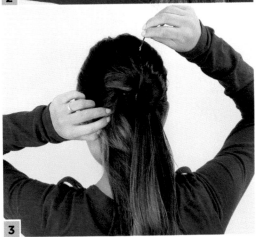

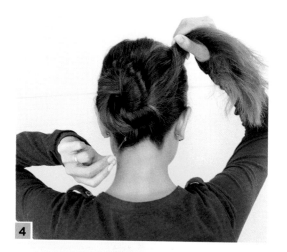

4. Wrap the twist around the base of the ponytail. Now pick up the bottom half of the ponytail (the part that was originally left down) so you can combine it with your twist. Gently comb through the loose hair at this point if it has started to get tangled. Twist all the hair together and begin wrapping the hair upwards for the second half of the infinity. Be sure to pin as you go so it maintains its shape.

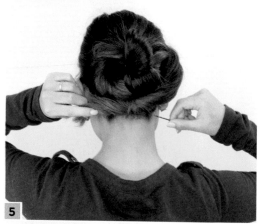

5. Now create the other side of the infinity symbol by wrapping the hair up towards the top of the head, then curving it back around, creating a backwards "C" shape, and wrapping the ends of the hair underneath the bottom of the infinity. Be sure to pin as you wrap so it stays in place.

6. If the hair is really long, wrap the twist back up the left side of the bun and tuck the tail underneath the twist to hide it before securing it with more bobby pins. Mist the entire style with hairspray to ensure that it holds throughout the entire day.

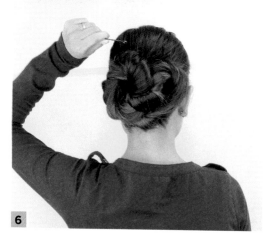

UPDO EXTRAS

When wrapping the hair around for the Infinity Bun, keep the twist tight and the bun small. It is easier to loosen the twist afterwards, and if you start the bun out too large there may not be enough hair left over to create the right side of the bun. Gently loosening the bun at the end will also help hide the bobby pins and the extra hair that is wrapped around the left side if you end up with a tail that is too long.

CHAPTER 3

Low Buns

A little fancier than your typical topknot or messy bun, the low updos in this chapter feature elegant styles with knots, braids, and wrapped buns that are perfect for a prom, a wedding, or a glamorous night out. It's easy to glam up a low bun by ensuring the top of the hair is smooth and polished for a sleeker style. Of course, they can be worn more casually for running errands and can even make hair that is due for a washing look suave. With beautiful styles like the Elegant Low Bun, Easy Loop Bun, and Wrapped Rolled Bun, you'll be feeling fabulous in no time!

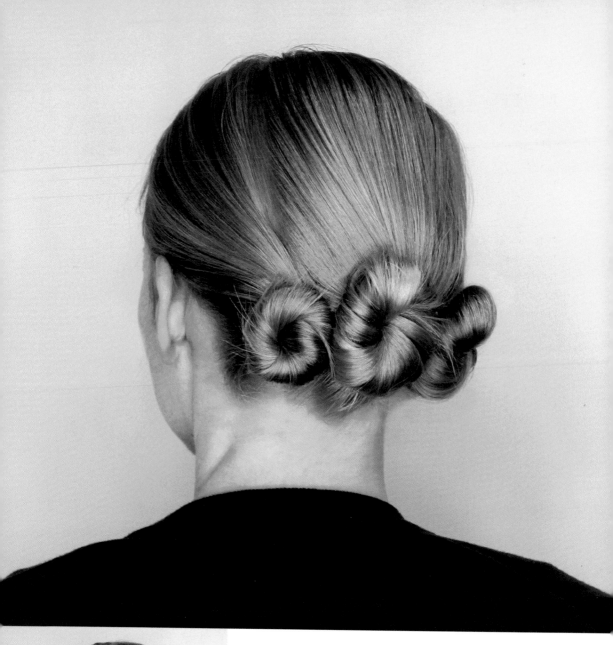

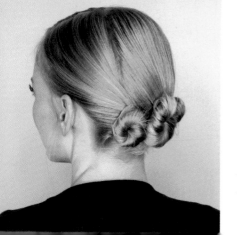

Three Twisted Buns

Three Twisted Buns is a great hairstyle for long, medium, or even shorter hair, and you can customize your look and wear this style super sleek or a little bit messy. Either way, it takes mere minutes to do and is a great style for days on the go. Get your hair up and out of the way with this cute hairstyle—keep it in your repertoire for days when you are rushing out the door, your hair is a tad too dirty to wear down, or just when you want to try something new!

MATERIALS

» Paddle brush
» Maximum-hold hairspray
» Wide-tooth comb
» 2 duck-bill clips
» 10–12 bobby pins

1. Begin by brushing through the hair to remove any tangles. Spray the hair with hairspray and comb through it once more to smooth down any flyaways. Next, create a part from the right corner of the crown down to the nape of the neck and clip off the front hair with a duck-bill clip.

2. Repeat the previous step on the left side by parting the hair from the left corner of the crown down to the nape of the neck and clipping it off with another duck-bill clip.

3. Take the loose center section of hair and twist it together.

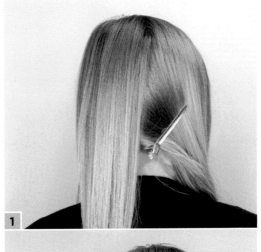

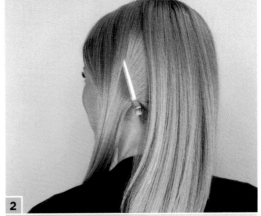

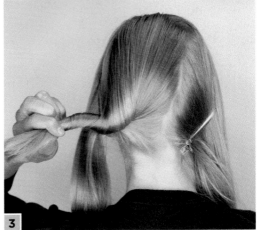

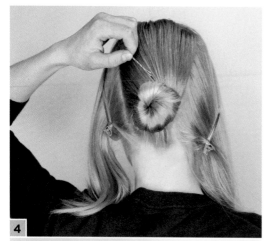

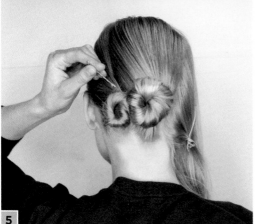

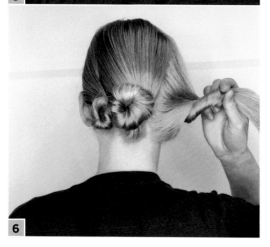

4. Wrap the twist around to create a tight bun at the nape of the neck. To ensure that the bun is secure, place one pin at each of the four "corners" of the bun and then spray the bun with hairspray.

5. Let down the hair clipped off on the left side and create a second bun, pinning it directly next to the middle bun. For a sleek bun, comb through the section first, then hairspray it and comb through it a second time to smooth down loose hairs before twisting it. Spray this bun with hairspray to ensure that it stays in place.

6. Let down the right section of hair and again twist the hair to create the third bun, first combing, spraying, and smoothing it as before.

7. Wrap the hair into a third bun and pin it in place with bobby pins, then mist the rest of the hair with hairspray to set the finished style.

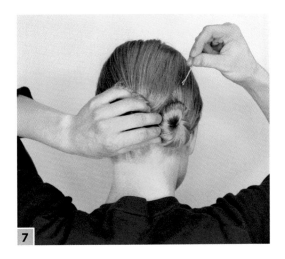

7

UPDO EXTRAS

To create a bit of volume at the top of the head, back-comb the hair at the start and smooth down the top layer before sectioning off the hair for the buns. For a looser look, gently pull on the edges of the buns to create volume and larger, looser buns.

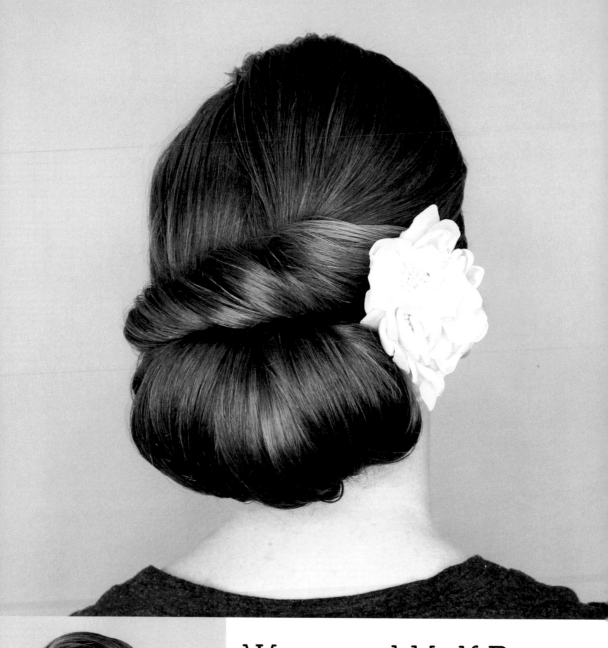

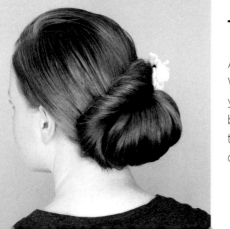

Wrapped Half Bun

A fancy updo that is both gorgeous and breathtaking, this Wrapped Half Bun looks tricky, but it isn't half as difficult as you might think. Take it in sections and you will be surprised by how simple it actually is. Wow the crowd with this beautiful low bun and be the belle of the ball at your next special occasion.

MATERIALS

» Wide-tooth comb
» 1 duck-bill clip
» 2 clear elastic bands
» Maximum-hold hairspray
» 5–6 bobby pins
» Clip or barrette (optional)

1. Comb through the hair to ensure there aren't any tangles. Next, separate off a portion of hair in a square pattern from the part, down the back of the head, level with the top of the ears, then across to the right ear. Clip off this section with a duck-bill clip to work with later.

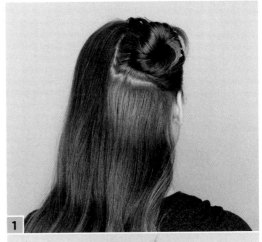

2. Comb the rest of the hair into a low ponytail, slightly off-center to the left, and secure it with a clear elastic band. To create a sleek and smooth style, spray the hair with hairspray before tying it up.

3. Next, create an upside-down topsy tail by gently loosening the ponytail, creating a gap just above the elastic, and flipping the tail up and through the gap.

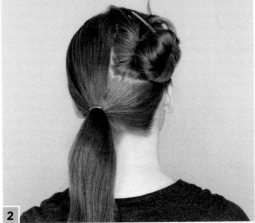

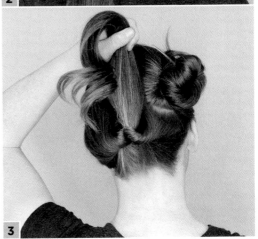

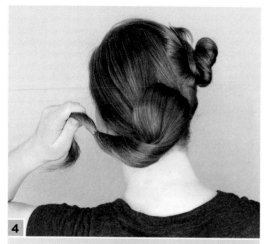

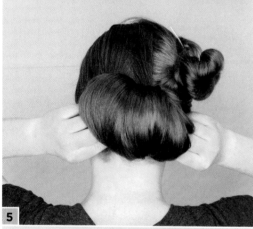

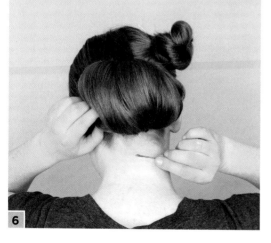

4. Comb through the tail of the ponytail, spray it with hairspray, and comb through it once more to ensure that it is smooth and free of flyaways. Then tie a clear elastic band near the end of the hair.

5. Roll the ponytail inwards and up towards the base, creating a thick rolled bun.

6. Pin down the bun by sliding bobby pins underneath it horizontally so they are hidden underneath the ponytail while holding it securely in place. Spray the bun with hairspray and glide a hand over the top to smooth down any loose hairs.

7. Let down the clipped portion of hair. Comb through it, mist it with hairspray, then comb through it once more before twisting the hair together in an upwards twist.

8. Lay the twist over the top of the bun, wrap it around the left side, and pin the end under the bun. Spray the finished 'do with hairspray so it stays in place. If desired, slide a pretty clip or barrette on the right side to dress up the look even more.

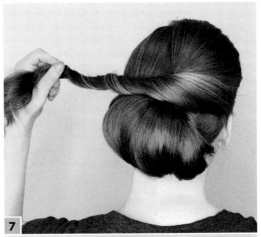

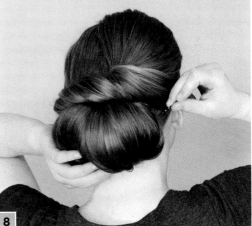

UPDO EXTRAS

Before and after each step, spray the hair with hairspray to ensure that the finished look is smooth and sleek. After laying the top twist over the bun, secure it with a bobby pin or two to ensure that it stays in place. If the bun begins to droop, secure it with more bobby pins. It won't matter how many you use because they will all stay hidden underneath the bun.

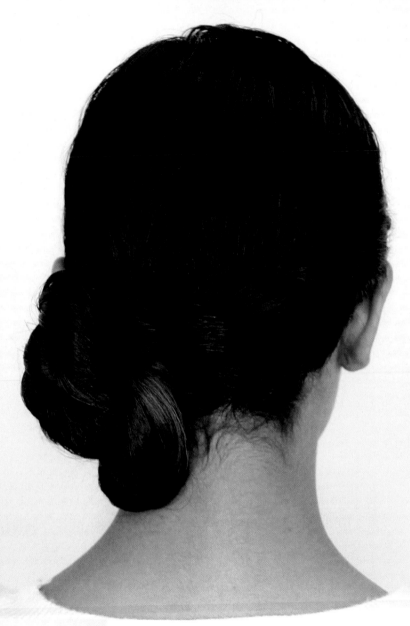

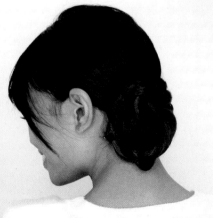

Rope Braid Bun

This Rope Braid Bun puts a fun new twist on the side bun. This hairstyle is one giant rope braid, all wrapped together to create a sleek style that is perfect for every single day. Wear it to work, to school, out on the town, or to lunch with friends. You will love it and they will too!

MATERIALS

» Wide-tooth comb
» 1 clear elastic band
» 4–6 bobby pins
» Maximum-hold hairspray

1. After combing through the hair, pick up a section right behind the right ear, from the part down to the nape of the neck.

2. Divide the section into two strands and twist the bottom section over the top section.

3. Pick up a new strand of hair and combine it with one of the original two strands, then twist the strands around each other once more.

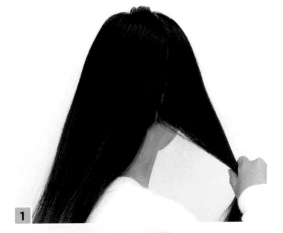

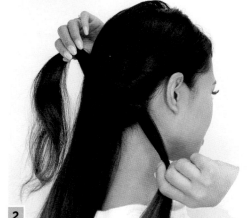

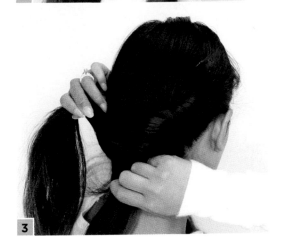

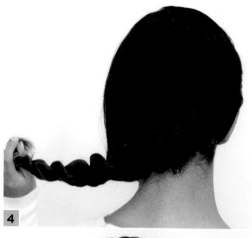

4. Continue twisting the strands together, bringing in small sections of new hair with each twist. When all the hair is brought in, continue twisting the hair until you reach the ends and have made a full-length rope braid. Tie off the end of the braid with a clear elastic band.

5. Wrap the rope braid into a low side bun, directly behind the left ear, at the nape of the neck. Pin down the bun with bobby pins, sliding them towards the center of the bun. Set the style with hairspray and smooth down any stray hairs.

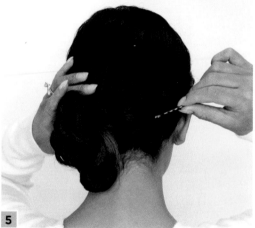

UPDO EXTRAS

Be sure to spray the hair with hairspray and comb through it before each twist. This will ensure that the hair stays untangled and will look smooth and sleek in the end.

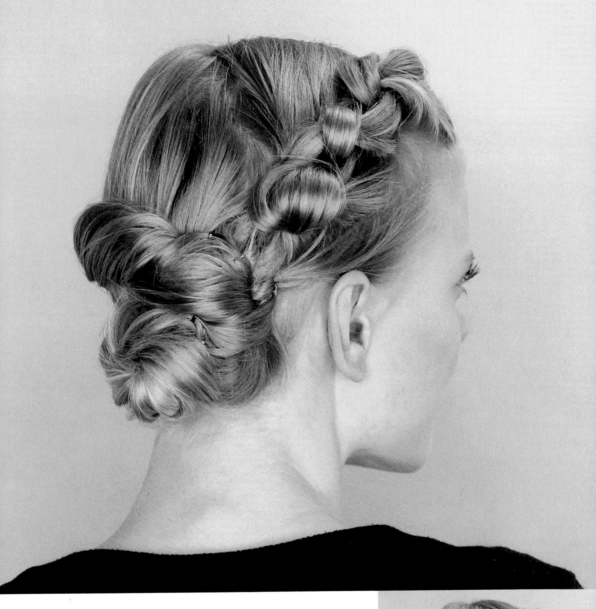

Knots and Low Bun

You may think of knotted hair as messy, but with the Knots and Low Bun it's okay to have your hair in knots—this hairstyle is literally created by tying it up. The bun at the back can be done a number of different ways. Try out this version first, then change it up depending on your mood. You can knot all the hair or just sweep it into a messy bun. See how it works for you and then surprise your friends with this unique everyday style.

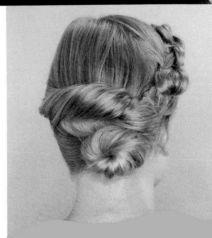

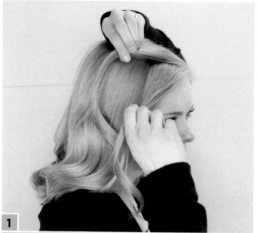

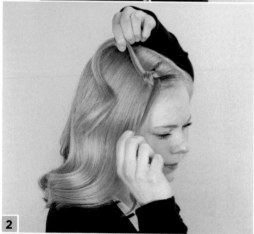

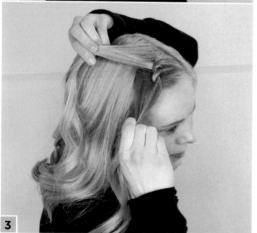

MATERIALS

» Wide-tooth comb
» 1 clear elastic band
» 6–8 bobby pins
» Maximum-hold hairspray

1. Comb through the hair to remove any tangles, then part the hair in a deep left-side part. Pick up a triangle shaped section, 2" back from the hairline and down to the temple on the right side. Divide this section into two strands.

2. Take the strand in the front into your left hand, and the strand in the back into your right hand. Then cross the strand in your left hand over the one in your right hand, creating a small hole. Loop the tail of the strand that is now in your right hand up and through the inside of the hole to create a half knot. Carefully pull the knot tight against the head.

3. Pick up a section of hair and add it into the left-hand strand. Then pick up another section of hair and add it to the right-hand strand for the next knot.

4. Cross the strands over each other and create a second knot with the strands. Gently pull it tight against the head.

5. Bring in more hair for each strand and create a third knot, pulling it tight again.

6. Tie off the knots with a clear elastic band.

7. Pick up a 1" section of hair above the left ear and twist the hair upwards, adding in hair as you go, twisting the piece towards the right side of the head.

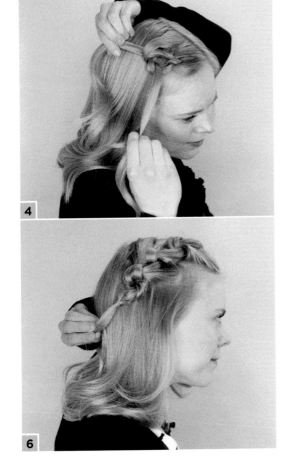

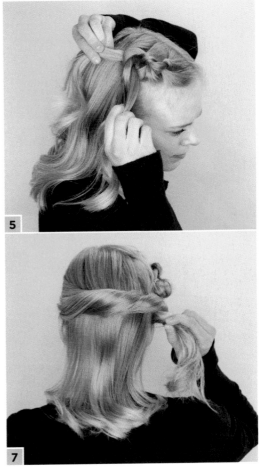

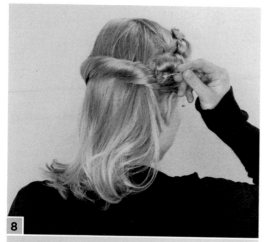

8

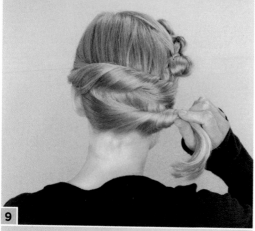

9

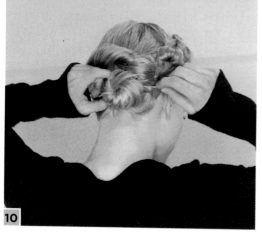

10

8. Lay the previously tied knots underneath the twist and pin the twist down directly behind the right ear, hiding the tail and elastic band of the knots.

9. Pick up the remaining hair and create another twist, rolling the hair upwards towards the right ear again.

10. Wrap the hair into a bun behind the right ear, and pin it in place with bobby pins. Slide the bobby pins towards the center of the bun so they are hidden. Liberally spray the style with hairspray to ensure it stays in place.

UPDO EXTRAS

After tying each knot, run a comb through the strands to ensure there are fewer tangles and flyaways. After creating the bun in Step 10, gently pull on the edges after it is pinned to create a more voluminous bun.

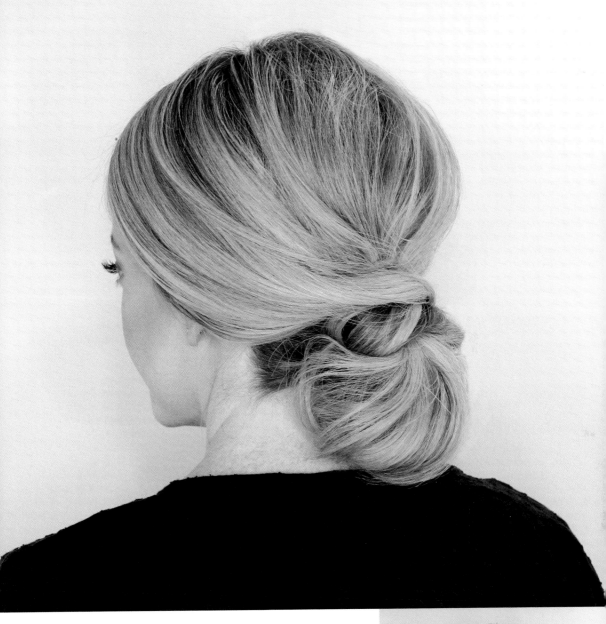

Elegant Low Bun

Dress up your low bun with this gorgeous style. It's a little retro, a little modern, and great for every day. The best part is that it is easy to create. Try out this Elegant Low Bun for your next event or even for just a lazy day at home and you will be wearing it more often than you think!

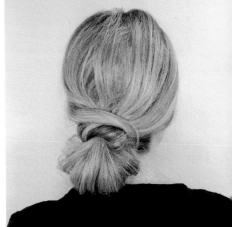

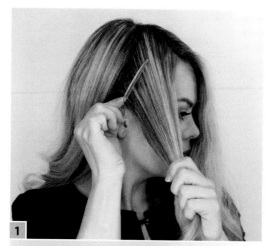

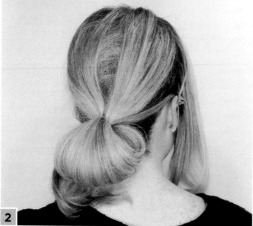

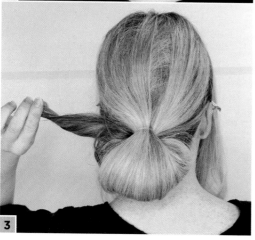

MATERIALS

> » 2 duck-bill clips
> » Paddle brush
> » 1 clear elastic band
> » 6–7 bobby pins
> » Medium-hold hairspray
> » Wide-tooth comb

1. Start with a part on the right side. Divide off a section of hair, 2" back from the hairline, down to the top of the right ear. Clip off the front section with a clip. Repeat this step on the left side, sectioning off a portion of hair from the part down to the top of the left ear, clipping off the front section.

2. Brush through the back section of hair to remove any tangles. Sweep the hair in this section into a low ponytail. Wrap a clear elastic band over the hair, creating a bun by pulling the hair halfway through on the last loop.

3. Pick up the end of the hair that didn't get pulled through the loop in the previous step and twist it together.

4. Wrap the twist around the hair elastic and continue wrapping until the entire piece is wrapped and you are holding the very end. Then pin down the end with a bobby pin. Be sure to hide the pin by sliding it into the hair, under the bun.

5. Take the hair that you previously pinned on the right side, spray it with hairspray, then comb through it to smooth it down. Lay the section over the top of the bun and wrap it counter-clockwise around the bun until you are holding the very end of the section.

6. Pin down the end of the wrapped piece to secure it around the bun.

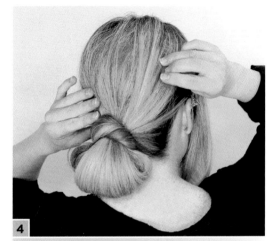

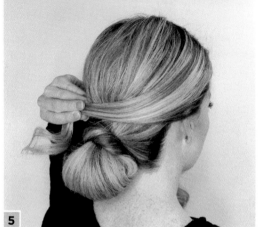

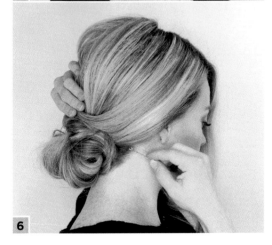

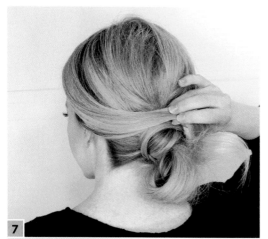

7

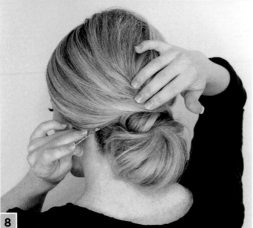

8

7. Take the hair that you previously pinned on the left side, spray it with hairspray, then comb through it to smooth it down. Drape this section over the top of the bun, as in the previous step, but wrap it clockwise around the bun, and continue wrapping until you are holding the very end.

8. Pin down the end of the wrapped piece to secure it around the bun. Liberally spray the style with hairspray and smooth your hands over the hair to lay down any loose hairs.

UPDO EXTRAS

For a more dramatic style, back-comb the hair at the beginning and smooth down the top layer of hair to cover it. After creating the bun, gently pull up the hair at the crown to create volume at the back.

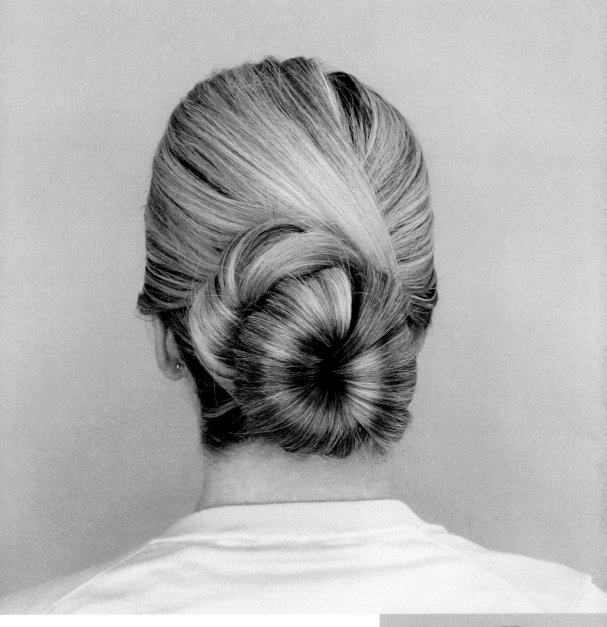

Double-Wrapped Bun

A bun is one of the most convenient hairstyles out there. A messy bun is perfect for when you are rushing out the door. This Double-Wrapped Bun is great when you want to feel a little more polished and put-together. It uses the basic technique behind the Donut Bun (in Chapter 1) but with a few extra wrapped pieces from the front, you will get a chic, new going-out hairstyle.

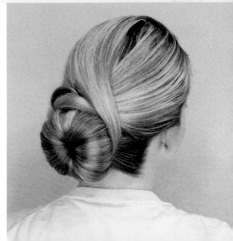

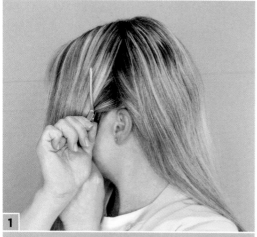

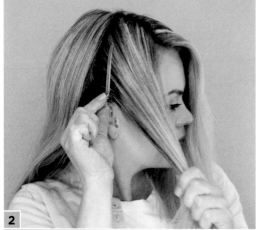

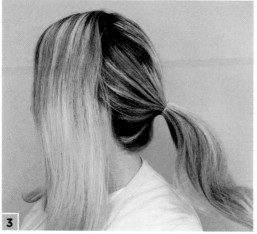

MATERIALS

- » 2 duck-bill clips
- » Wide-tooth comb
- » 2 clear elastic bands
- » Hair donut
- » 4–6 bobby pins
- » Maximum-hold hairspray

1. Separate off a portion of hair from the part down to the left ear and clip the front portion out of the way using a duck-bill clip.

2. Repeat the previous step on the other side. You'll wrap these two front sections around the bun at the end.

3. Comb through the rest of the hair and sweep it up into a ponytail slightly lower than ear level. Secure it with a clear elastic band.

4. Slide a hair donut over the ponytail.

5. Lean your head forward and spread the ponytail around the hair donut so it evenly covers it. Then wrap a clear elastic band over the bun to hold it in place.

6. Take any hair that sticks out from the bun and wrap it around the base of the bun, then pin it down with bobby pins. Slide the pins into the center of the bun so they remain hidden.

7. Let down the clipped hair on the right side and comb through it to smooth it down. Spray the strands with hairspray, then comb through them once more to smooth down flyaways.

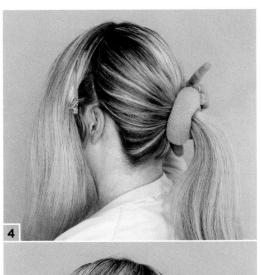

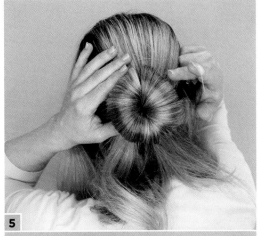

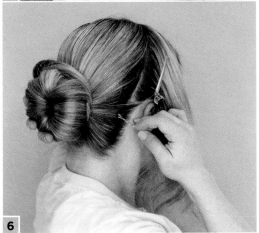

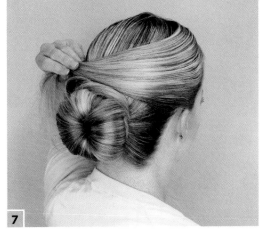

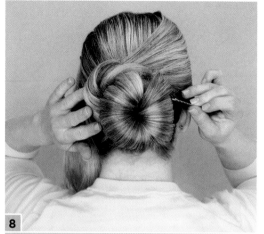

8

8. Bring the hair across the top of the bun, then wrap it around the bun counter-clockwise. Pin down the ends, sliding the pins into the bun to hide them.

9. Let down the pinned hair on the left side and comb through it to smooth it down. Spray the strands with hairspray then comb through them once more to smooth down flyaways. Bring the hair across the top of the bun, then wrap it around the bun clockwise.

10. Pin down the ends, sliding the pins into the bun to hide them. Then set the style with hairspray to ensure it stays in place all day.

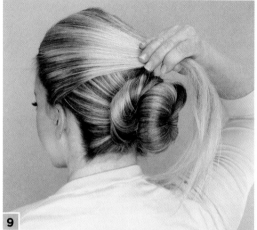

9

UPDO EXTRAS

If you part the hair on the side, one of the front portions will be thicker than the other. Wrap the thin side first, then wrap the thicker side over the top. To guarantee a sleek finish, run a comb through the strands, mist them with hairspray, and comb through them once more before each step.

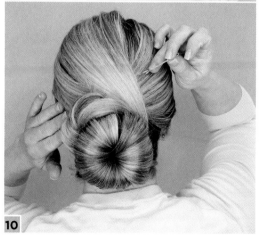

10

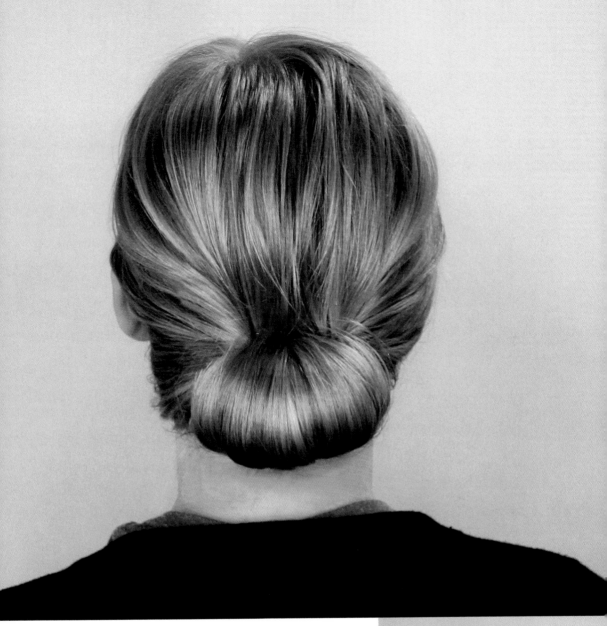

Low Tucked Bun

A super cute low bun, this Low Tucked Bun looks sleek and easy—because it is! The trick is all in the flipped loop, or topsy tail, whichever name you prefer. If you want to make this structured bun look a little more casual, all you have to do is back-comb the ponytail before tucking it for a lived-in feel. Sleek, structured, and totally customizable? What's not to love!

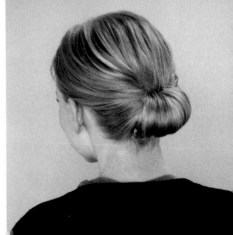

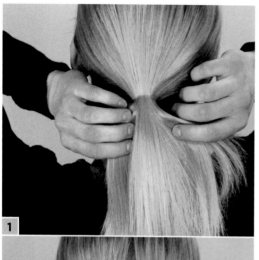

MATERIALS

» Wide-tooth comb
» 1 clear elastic band
» Medium-hold hairspray
» 4–6 bobby pins

1. Comb all of the hair into a low ponytail and secure it with a clear elastic band. Be sure to spray the hair with hairspray as you comb it to reduce the flyaways and create a smooth ponytail.

2. Use your fingers to create a gap right above the elastic band, separating the hair in half.

3. Flip the ponytail up and through the gap, pulling it back down tight to create a topsy tail.

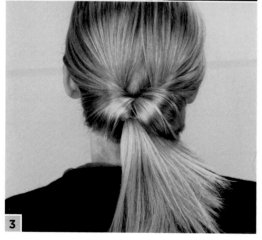

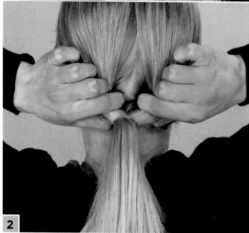

4. Reach into the top of the gap previously made and pull the ponytail halfway out, as if undoing the previous tucking. This will create a round bun shape but ensure the ends of the hair stay hidden behind the bun.

5. Slide some pins vertically into the top of the bun to secure it against the head. Then set the style with hairspray and smooth down any stray hairs.

UPDO EXTRAS

After creating the ponytail, back-comb the underside of the ponytail, before flipping it through the topsy tail in Step 3, to add a bit of volume to the finished bun.

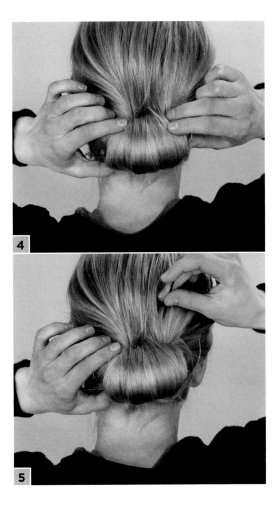

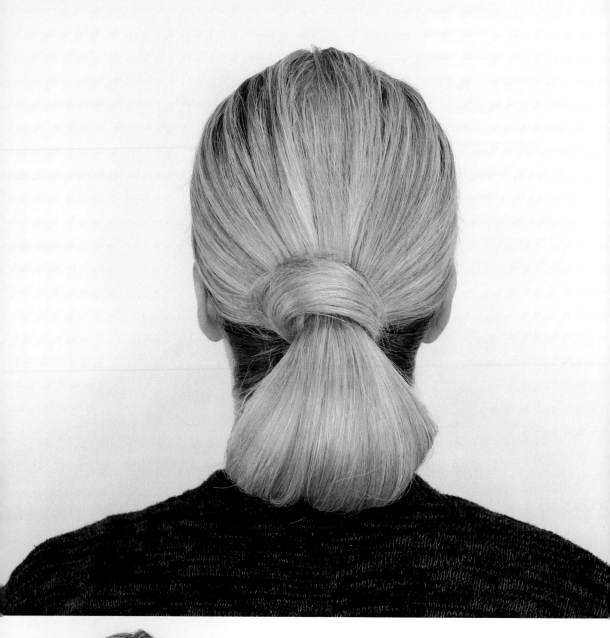

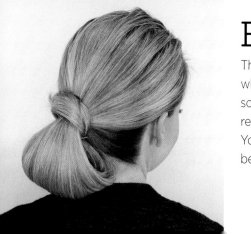

Easy Loop Bun

This Easy Loop Bun is a super quick and easy style for days when you're on the run or when you're just ready to try something new. With no braiding or intricate handiwork required, this simple bun will literally take you seconds to do. You will be so glad you have this in your beauty repertoire because it really is as easy as it looks!

MATERIALS

» Wide-tooth comb
» Maximum-hold hairspray
» 1 clear elastic band
» 2-3 bobby pins

1. Comb all the hair straight back, then mist it with hairspray and sweep it up into a ponytail that sits slightly below the ears.

2. Secure the ponytail by wrapping a clear elastic once over the hair, pulling the hair all the way through the band.

3. Wrap the clear elastic around the ponytail a second time, but only pull the hair halfway through to create a loop.

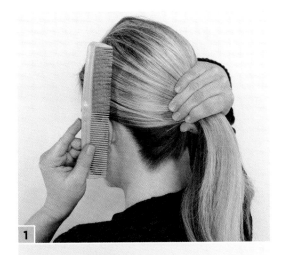

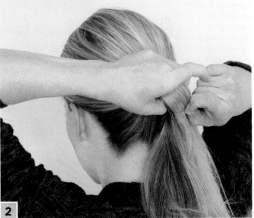

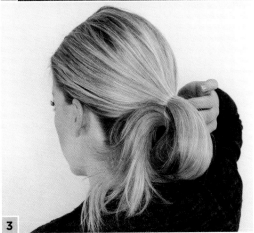

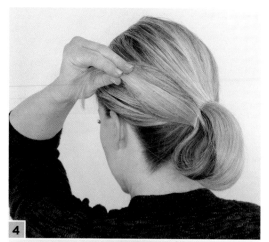

4. Pick up the ends of the hair and wrap them around the elastic band.

5. Pin the end of the wrapped hair by sliding the pin towards the center of the ponytail so it is hidden. Finally, mist the entire style with hairspray so it stays in place.

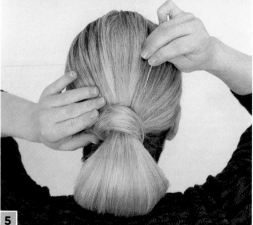

UPDO EXTRAS

For a smaller bun, pull the hair a third of the way through the elastic on the second wrap so the loop is smaller. After creating the loop, spray it with hairspray and run your hand over the bun to smooth down any stray hairs.

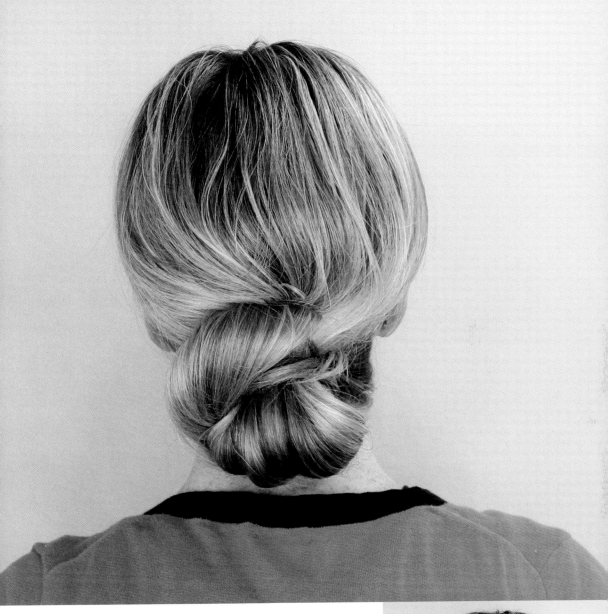

Low Twisted Bun

This gorgeous bun is so easy to do you won't believe it! It's a hairstyle that will find a permanent place in your beauty arsenal, the type of bun that you will return to over and over again. It is perfect for all hair types and can be styled to create a bigger or smaller bun depending on your preference.

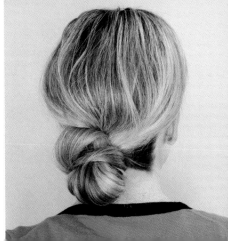

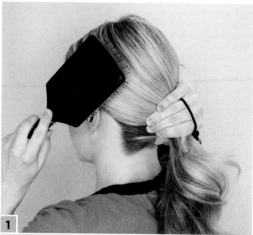

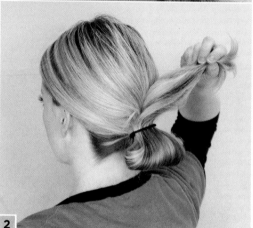

MATERIALS

» Paddle brush
» Medium-hold hairspray
» 1 hair hairband
» 3–4 bobby pins

1. Brush the hair into a low ponytail. Remove any tangles and smooth down any flyaways with hairspray.

2. Wrap the hair with a hairband, creating a bun by pulling the hair halfway through on the last loop so the ends face upwards.

3. Wrap the ends around the hairband and pin the ends with bobby pins.

4. Gently pull the hair loose at the back of the head to create volume, then mist the hair with hairspray and smooth down any last loose hairs.

UPDO EXTRAS

Create extra volume by back-combing the hair at the crown before getting started, then smooth down the top layer to hide the teased portion. Also, when wrapping the hair for the bun create a smaller bun at first, because it can always be made larger later on.

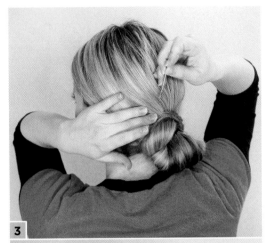

3

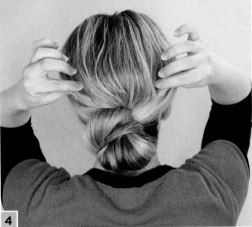

4

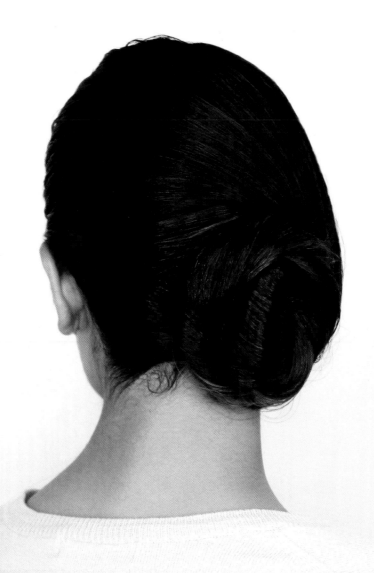

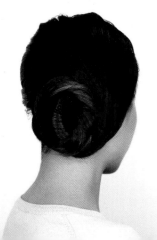

Wrapped Rolled Bun

This Wrapped Rolled Bun is a glamorous side bun that is intricately wrapped and perfect for that special occasion. Wear it on your next date or save it for an upcoming wedding or party. You will definitely wow the crowd with this one.

MATERIALS

» Wide-tooth comb
» 1–2 duck-bill clips
» 1 clear elastic band
» 6–8 bobby pins
» Maximum-hold hairspray

1. Separate the hair into two sections from the top of the ears to the back of the head, and secure the top section with 1–2 duck-bill clips, depending on the hair thickness.

2. Sweep the bottom section into a low, off-center ponytail that sits below the right ear, and tie it off with a clear elastic band.

3. Twist the ponytail and wrap it into a bun around the elastic band. Then secure it in place with bobby pins.

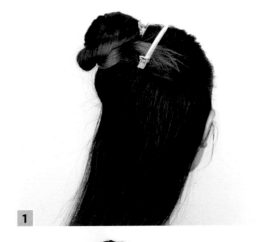

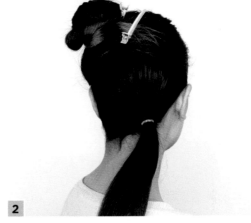

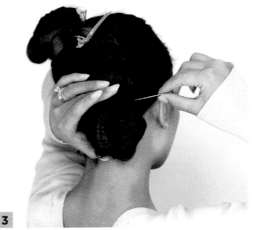

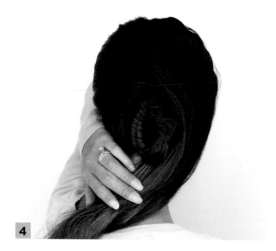

4. Let down the top portion that was previously pinned and wrap it around the right side of the bun.

5. Continue wrapping the section clockwise around the bun until you reach the end of the hair. Pin down the end with bobby pins. Use as many as you need so the bun feels tight against the head, and be sure to hide the pins underneath the bun. Then set the style with hairspray and smooth down any stray hairs.

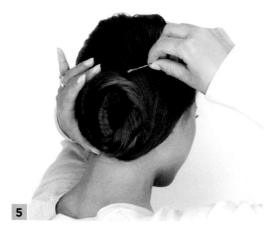

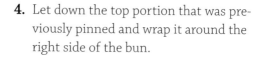

UPDO EXTRAS

Always brush through the hair before beginning any style to smooth it down and remove any tangles. Also, brush through the top portion of hair before wrapping it around the bun. This will ensure that it lies smoothly and will prevent any bumps or snarls.

CHAPTER 4

Braided Updos

In this chapter you'll learn how to embellish any bun with a pretty braid. Whether you are using a regular braid, trying your hand at a French or Dutch braid, or mastering the trendy fishtail braid, all it takes is a bit of practice whenever you have a free moment. The more you practice, the better you will get, and the more intricate the braid, the more amped up your style will become! To achieve that extra wow factor with your braids, loosen and flatten them out by gently pulling on the edges. You'll never look at braids the same way again!

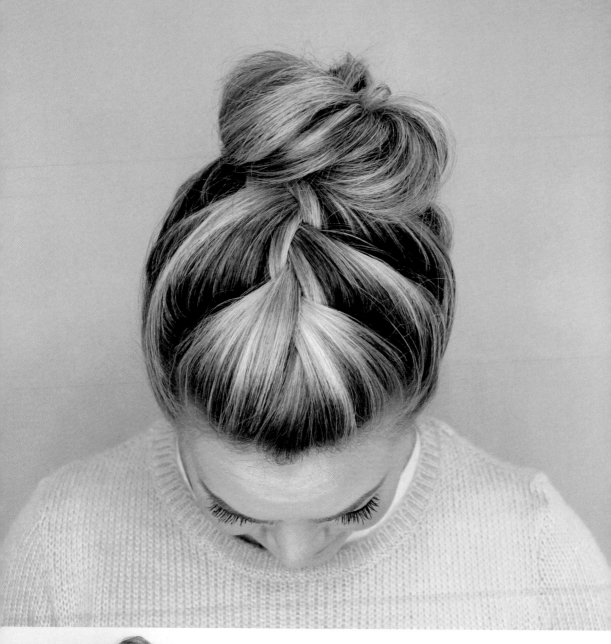

French Braid High Bun

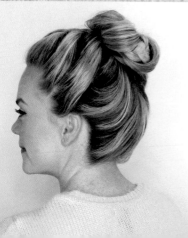

Top off your topknot with a chic French braid. Adding a cool braid along the top of the head is easy to do and is a great way to make your everyday bun look more fun and polished. Create the braid first and end it where you normally wear your bun. You can even switch out a typical, everyday bun for any of your favorites. Try it out with the Cotton Candy Bun or Donut Bun, in particular!

MATERIALS

» Paddle brush
» Maximum-hold hairspray
» Wide-tooth comb
» 1 clear elastic band
» 4–6 bobby pins

1. Start by brushing the hair straight back so it's smooth. Separate out a section of hair at the hairline that runs the width of the forehead. Spray this section with hairspray, then comb through it so it is smooth.

2. Carefully divide this section of hair into three equal strands for the French braid portion.

3. Begin a French braid by crossing the strand on the left over the middle strand.

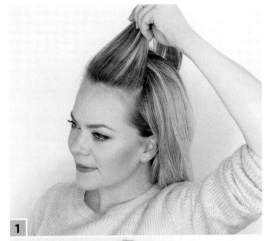

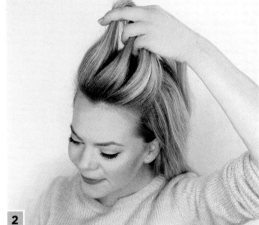

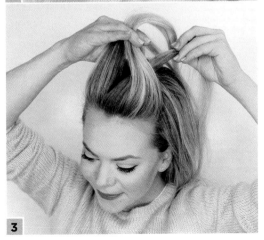

4. Now cross the right-side strand over the middle strand.

5. Pick up a section of hair and incorporate it into the left-side strand. Now cross this section over the middle strand. Incorporating sections of hair into the strands will create the French braid, so be sure to bring in hair every time to ensure that the braid is even on both sides.

6. Continue bringing in sections and braiding the hair until it reaches the spot where you will place your bun.

7. Braid the rest of this section into a regular braid and tie it off with a clear elastic band so it doesn't come loose and slip out.

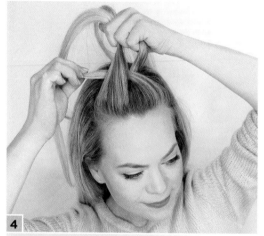

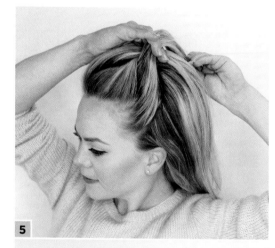

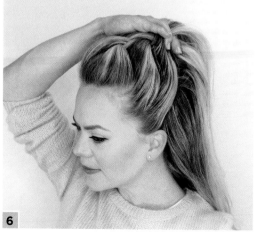

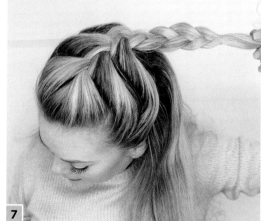

8. Sweep all the hair, including the tail of the braid, into a high ponytail at the back of the crown. Spray the underside of the hair with hairspray and run a comb through it to ensure all the tangles are removed and the flyaways are smoothed down.

9. Twist all the hair together to create the bun portion. At this point you can remove the clear elastic band from the end of the braid but be sure to keep a tight grip on the hair so the braid doesn't fall loose when wrapping the bun.

10. Wrap the hair around to create a bun and pin it in place with bobby pins. I like to use at least four pins, pinning the "corners" of the bun so I know it is secure. Using four or more pins will ensure that the style is tight and will stay in place all day. Mist the entire style with hairspray and smooth down any loose hairs.

UPDO EXTRAS

When creating the French braid, pull in small sections of hair for a more detailed braid. If you are having trouble creating a tight style with the bun, secure the ponytail with an elastic band before wrapping it into the bun. Then, after securing the bun, gently pull on the edges to create a fuller, more voluminous look.

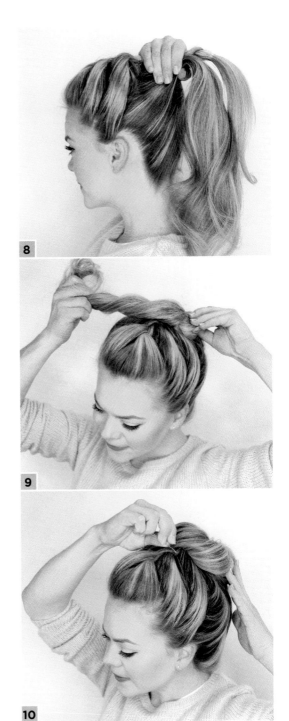

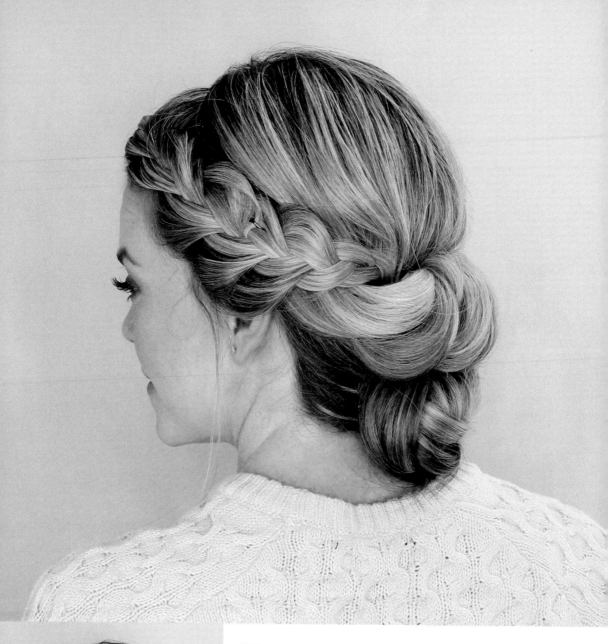

French Braid
Looped Bun

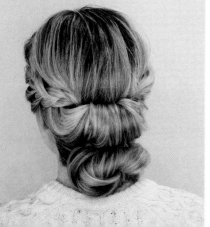

This hairstyle has it all: A French braid, looped headband, and wrapped bun, all tied together to create a chic new look that seems more complicated than it really is. This French Braid Looped Bun works best on second-day hair, but you can give clean hair a little bit of texture with a few spritzes of dry shampoo. Add some curls beforehand to help create a seamless style.

MATERIALS

- » Wide-tooth comb
- » 1 duck-bill clip
- » Stretchy headband
- » 4–6 bobby pins
- » 1 clear elastic band
- » Maximum-hold hairspray

1. Use a comb to separate a section of hair, from the part down to the left ear. Clip off the front portion with a duck-bill clip.

2. Place a stretchy headband over the center of the head, sliding the back portion down the back of the head at the nape of the neck. If the headband comes loose or pops off, pin it down with some bobby pins, sliding them over the band and downwards towards the neck.

3. Let down the front portion of hair and create a French braid by picking up a 1" section near the hairline and dividing it into three equal sections. Cross the left-side section over the middle section then the right-side section over the middle section. Pick up a section of hair, adding it into the left-side section and cross it over the middle section. Now pick up a section of hair, adding it into the right-side section and cross it over the middle section. Continue braiding, incorporating hair into the braid until it reaches the left ear. Then continue braiding this section down into a regular braid and tie off the end with a clear elastic band.

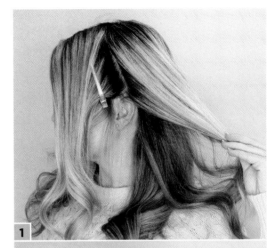

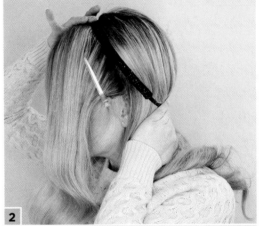

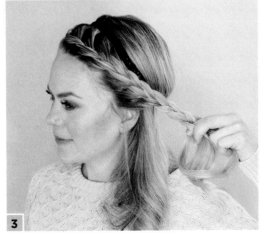

4. Wrap the braid around the headband, pulling it back down towards the neck.

5. Pick up a section of hair, directly underneath the braid, and wrap it around the headband as well, following along the braid.

6. Take a section of hair on the right side, near the face, and wrap it around the headband.

7. Pick up a section of hair, at the back of the head directly under the headband, and wrap it around the headband, tucking in the ends. Spray the roll with hairspray and smooth down any stray hairs.

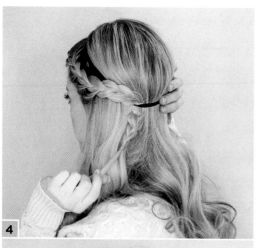

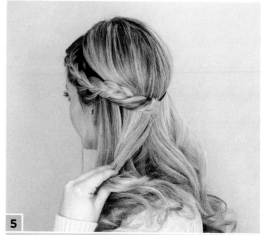

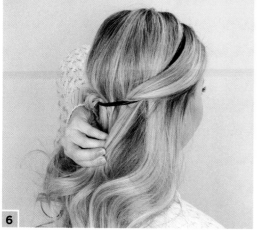

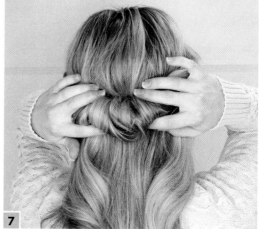

8. Pick up the remaining hair and twist it together.

9. Wrap the twist clockwise into a bun and pin it down with bobby pins. Hide the pins under the bun by sliding them towards the center. Then set the style with hairspray while smoothing a hand over the bun to smooth any stray hairs.

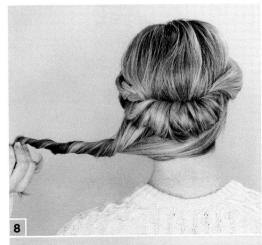

UPDO EXTRAS

Back-comb the hair at the crown to create a bit of volume. Run a comb over the top layer to ensure that the teased portion is hidden. You can also gently pull on the edges of the braid to make it fuller. Be sure to wrap the hair for the bun tighter at the beginning. It will naturally loosen after it's pinned, but you can also make it larger by gently pulling on the edges.

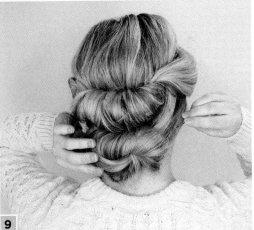

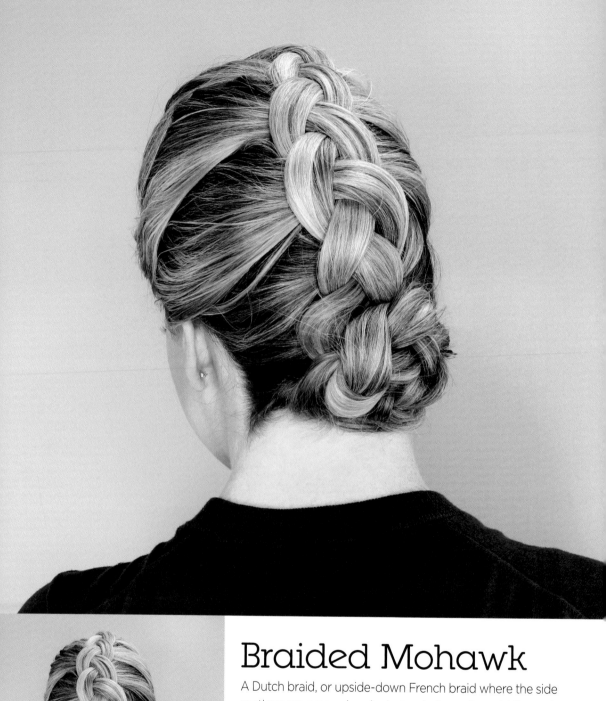

Braided Mohawk

A Dutch braid, or upside-down French braid where the side sections are crossed under instead of over the middle section, wrapped into a bun is a style that can be created to look smooth and sleek or loose and messy. It all depends on the occasion or event. This style works best with second-day hair but can be done on clean hair if you add a bit of texture with dry shampoo or spray wax. It is a great style for all hair types, too!

MATERIALS

» Paddle brush
» Maximum-hold hairspray
» 6–8 bobby pins
» 1 clear elastic band

1. Brush through the hair to smooth it out and remove any snarls. Pick up a section of hair at the corners of the forehead, separating it off from the rest. Brush through it to smooth it down and spritz it with hairspray.

2. Slightly twist the separated section so the left side wraps over the right side.

3. Slide a pin over the twist and push it in towards the face. This will hide the pin under the hair, while also holding the hair tightly in place.

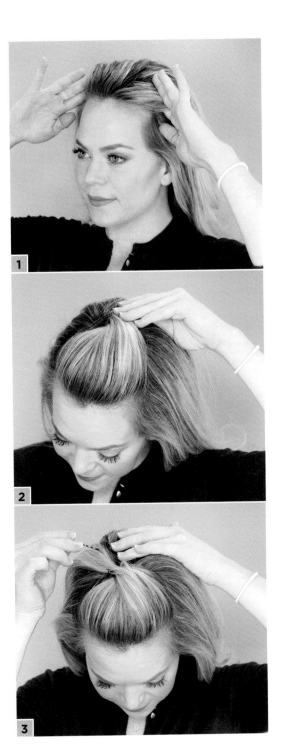

4. Separate out a portion of hair, halfway between the pinned portion and the ears.

5. Divide this section into three strands. Cross the right strand under the middle, then cross the left strand under the middle.

6. Cross the right strand under the middle and bring in a section of hair, crossing it under as well, incorporating it into the strand.

7. Continue braiding the hair down towards the nape of the neck, bringing in sections of hair with each cross-under.

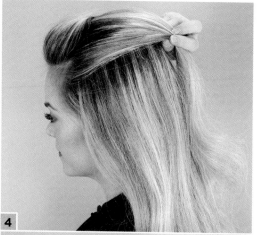

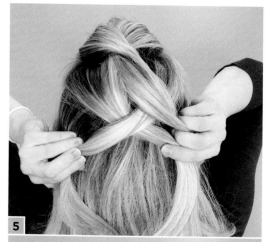

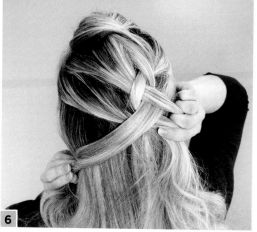

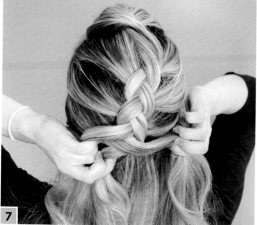

8. When all the hair is brought in, braid the rest of the hair down into a regular braid and tie off the end with a clear elastic band.

9. Wrap the tail of the braid counter-clockwise into a bun and secure the edges with bobby pins. Use as many as you need to make it feel snug and secure, but slide the pins under the hair so they stay out of view. Smooth down any stray hairs with hairspray and spritz the style to set it.

UPDO EXTRAS

Keep a firm grip on the three sections of hair as you braid it. If you let one side fall loose then the entire style will be loose in that spot at the end.

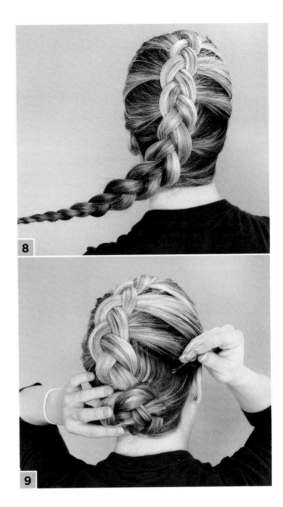

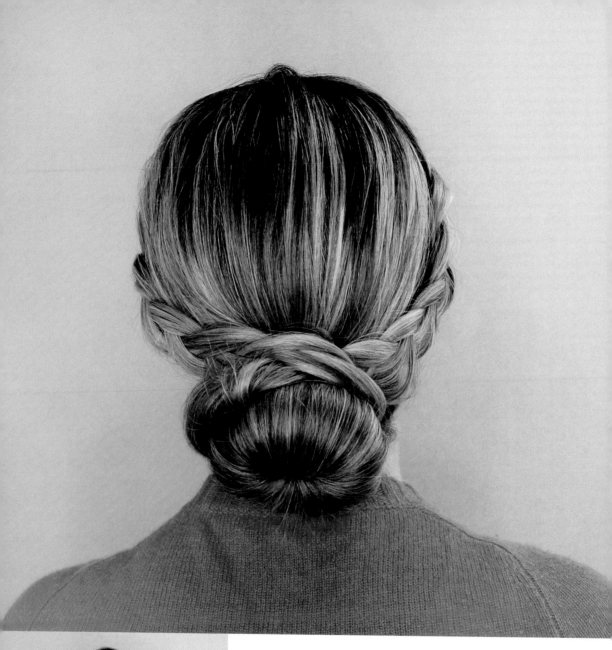

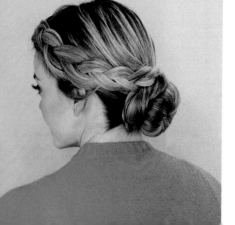

Side Braids and Bun

A sleek updo, embellished with two pretty braids, this style is perfect on second-day hair and works well on all hair types. Throw some curls into the hair beforehand to make creating the bun a little easier. Wear this style to work, or when hanging out with friends, or even for a special occasion; whatever suits your fancy suits this Side Braids and Bun!

MATERIALS

» Paddle brush
» 2 duck-bill clips
» Maximum-hold hairspray
» 1 hairband
» Hair donut
» 1 clear elastic band
» 3–4 bobby pins

1. Brush through the hair to smooth it out and remove any tangles. Then section off a portion of hair from the part down to the right ear and clip this section off with a duck-bill clip. Repeat on the left side.

2. Brush through the back portion of hair, spray it with hairspray, and brush it into a low ponytail. Tie it off with a hairband. It should sit lower than the ears, near the nape of the neck.

3. Place a hair donut over the ponytail so it sits at the base, over the elastic.

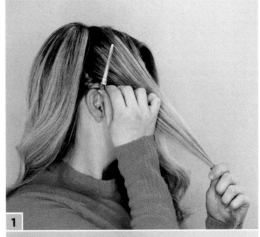

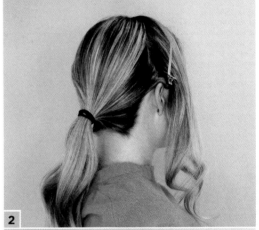

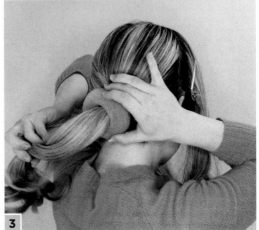

4. Spread the ponytail around the hair donut and pop a clear elastic band over the top to hold the hair in place.

5. Twist together the hair that hangs out from the bun.

6. Wrap the twist clockwise around the base of the bun and pin down the end.

7. Let down the clipped portion of hair on the right side and divide this section into three strands to create a Dutch braid. Cross the right strand under the middle, then cross the left strand under the middle. Then cross the right strand under the middle and bring in a new section of hair, crossing it under as well, incorporating it into the strand. Continue braiding

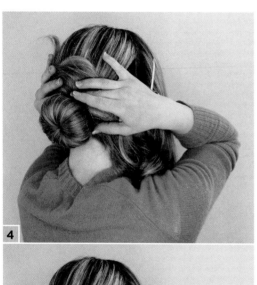

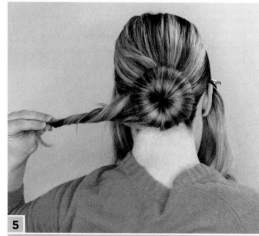

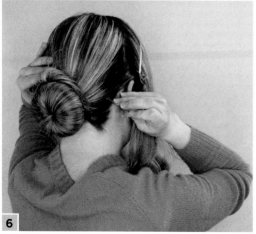

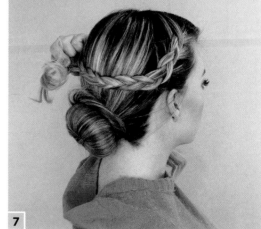

the hair, bringing in new sections of hair with each cross-under. When all the hair is brought in, braid the rest of the hair down into a regular braid.

8. Lay the braid over the bun, wrap it counter-clockwise around the bun, and pin down the end with a bobby pin.

9. Create a second Dutch braid with the clipped hair on the left side.

10. Wrap this braid clockwise around the bun, pinning down the end. Then smooth down any stray hairs with hairspray and spritz the style to set it.

UPDO EXTRAS

After banding the hair into a ponytail, brush through it and spray with hairspray, then brush through it once more to smooth down flyaways and create a sleek, finished bun. To finish the style, carefully pull on the edges of each braid to make them slightly fuller.

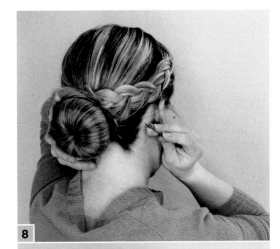

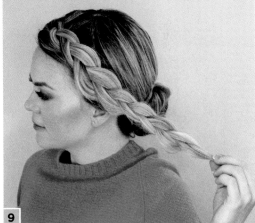

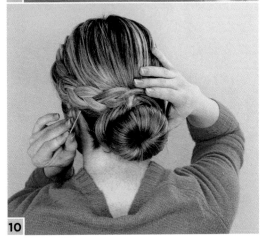

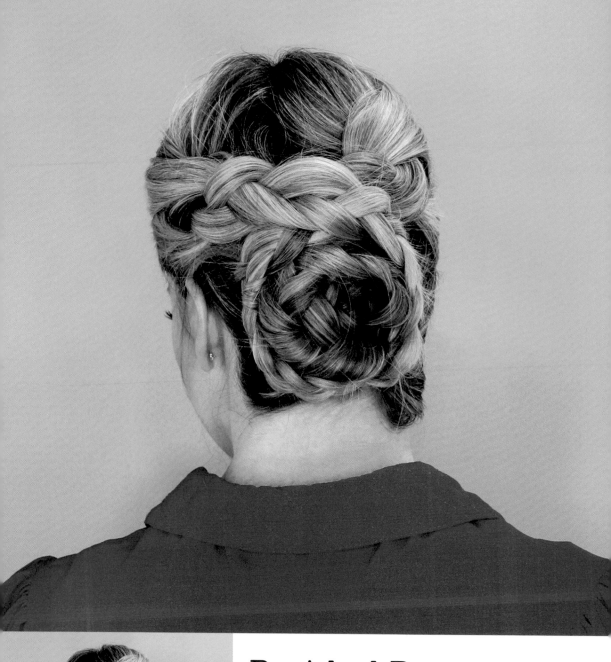

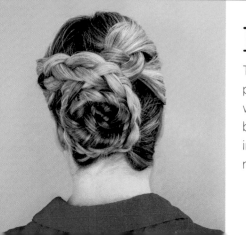

Braided Bun

This Braided Bun is a pretty updo that looks more complicated than it actually is, which is perfect for those times when you want to impress! It is made up of three regular braids all wrapped together so there isn't any tricky braiding at all. This lovely 'do is perfect for the office, for a formal night out, or even just for fun! So, let's get to it.

MATERIALS

- » Paddle brush
- » 3 clear elastic bands
- » 8–10 bobby pins
- » Maximum-hold hairspray

1. Brush through the hair to remove any tangles then part the hair either in the middle or on the side; either works fine. Pick up the section of hair from the part down to the left ear. Braid the section into a regular braid and tie off the end with a clear elastic band.

2. Create a second braid on the right side, using the hair from the part down to the right ear. Tie off this braid with another clear elastic band.

3. Create a third braid with the remaining hair and tie off the end with a third clear elastic band.

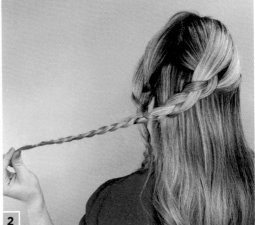

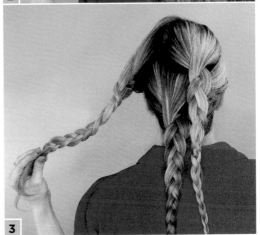

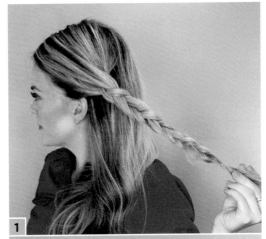

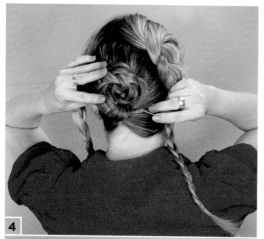

4. Wrap the bottommost braid into a bun and pin down the end with a bobby pin. Slide the pin under the bun so it stays out of view.

5. Pick up the right-side braid, lay it over the top of the bun, and wrap it counter-clockwise around the bun, pinning down the end with a bobby pin.

6. Now wrap the left-side braid over and then clockwise around the bun, pinning down the end. Set the style with hair-spray to ensure that it stays in place.

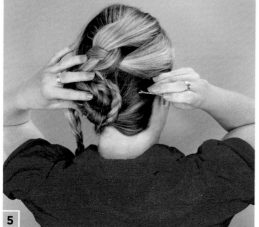

UPDO EXTRAS

After braiding each section, spray the braid with hairspray and slide a hand down the braid to smooth any stray hairs. Feel free to use as many pins as you need to ensure that the style is tight and won't fall out during the day.

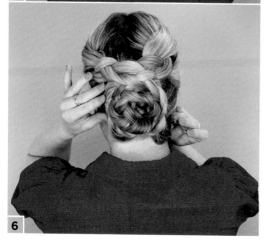

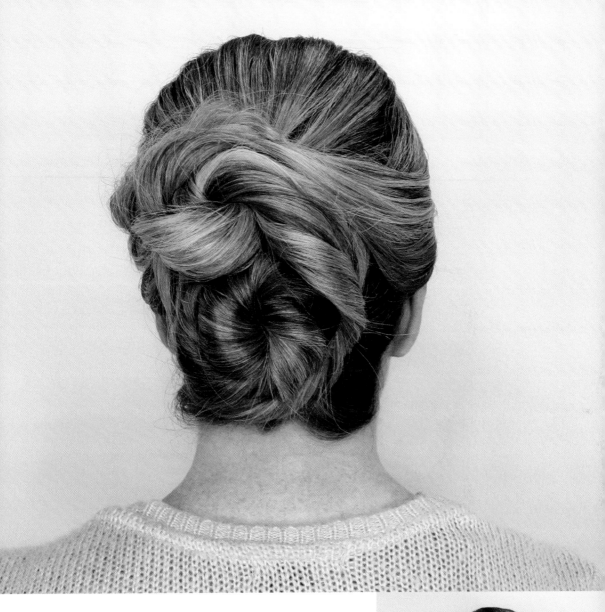

Inverted Fishtail Updo

The fishtail braid is the hottest braid right now, and this sleek Inverted Fishtail Updo featuring a Dutch fishtail braid, or upside-down fishtail braid, is super chic and a perfect way to look right on trend. If you've never worn a fishtail braid or don't know how to do one, then this tutorial is perfect for you!

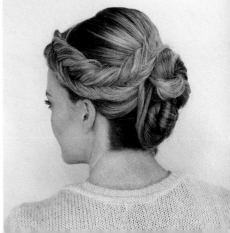

MATERIALS

- » Wide-tooth comb
- » 2 duck-bill clips
- » 3 clear elastic bands
- » 10–12 bobby pins
- » Maximum-hold hairspray

1. Comb through the hair, then divide off a portion from a side part down to the ear, clipping off the back section with a duck-bill clip.

2. Separate off a small portion of hair, near the part, of this front section.

3. Divide this new section into two halves, left and right.

4. Take a small piece from the right side, cross it underneath, and add it into the left side.

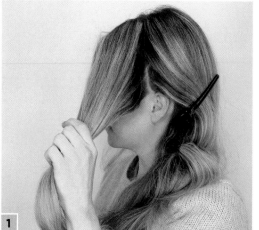

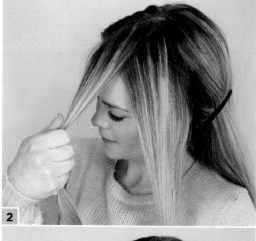

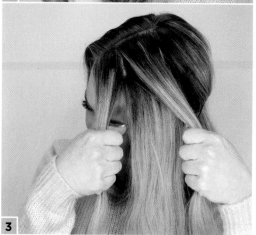

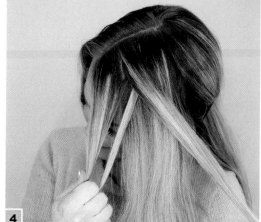

5. Now cross a small piece from the left side underneath, and add it into the right side.

6. Separate off another small piece from the right side. Bring in a new section of hair, add it to this piece, and cross both underneath, adding them into the section on the left.

7. Repeat the previous step with hair on the left: separate off a small piece of hair, pick up a new section, and cross both underneath to the right side.

8. Continue braiding this way to create a Dutch fishtail braid (or upside-down fishtail braid when the braid sits on top of the head).

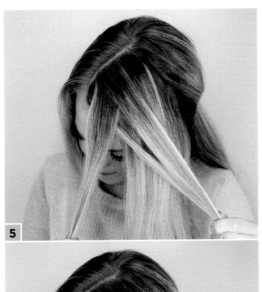

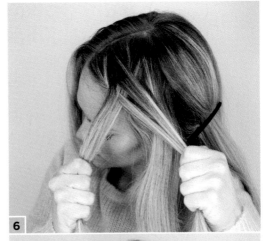

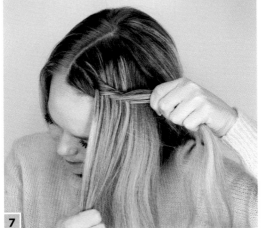

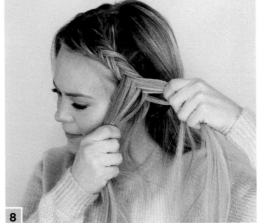

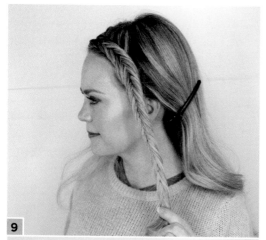

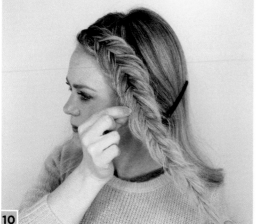

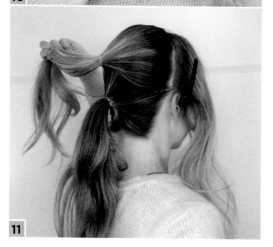

9. Once all the hair is brought into the braid, continue braiding the rest of the section into a fishtail braid. To do this, separate off a small section of hair from one side, cross it underneath and add it into the opposite side. Then separate off a small section from the other side, cross it underneath and add it into the opposite side.

10. Once the hair is braided, gently pull on the sides of the braid, carefully loosening them, to create a fuller, flatter braid. Then secure the end with an elastic band.

11. Separate off another section of hair from the part down to the right ear, clipping off the front portion with a duck-bill clip. Divide the remaining hair into two sections and tie each one into a ponytail with a clear elastic band.

12. Clip the top ponytail with a duck-bill clip so it's out of the way. Twist the bottom ponytail together and wrap it into a bun, securing it with bobby pins.

13. Let down the top ponytail and divide it into two sections. Clip off the top half using a duck-bill clip.

14. Twist the bottom section together and wrap it clockwise around the base of the clear elastic band and then around the bottom bun. Secure the end with bobby pins.

15. Unclip the top half of the ponytail, twist it together, and, following the first twist, wrapping it clockwise around the two buns as well.

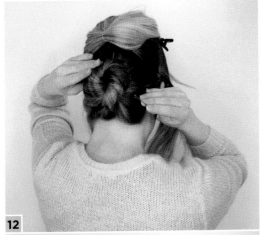

12

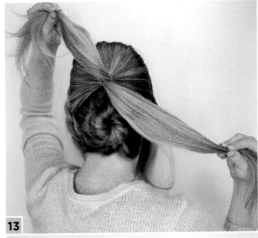

13

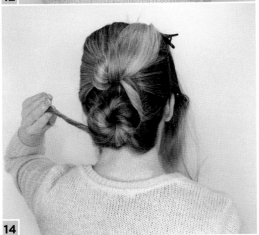

14

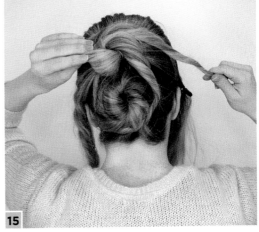

15

16. Pin down the end with bobby pins and secure any loose pieces.

17. Let down the pinned hair on the right side and comb through it to smooth out any tangles. Drape the section over the buns and wrap it counter-clockwise, securing the end with bobby pins.

18. Now drape the fishtail braid over the top of the bun, tucking the tail underneath the bun.

19. Pin down the end of the fishtail braid and any other sections that feel loose. Then set the entire style with a mist of hairspray and smooth your fingers over the sections to smooth down any loose hairs.

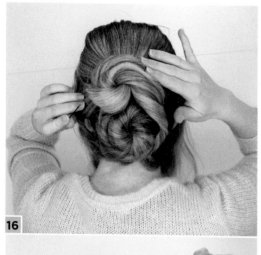

16

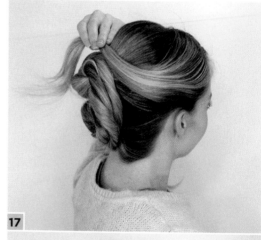

17

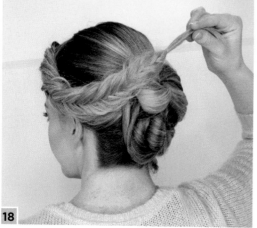

18

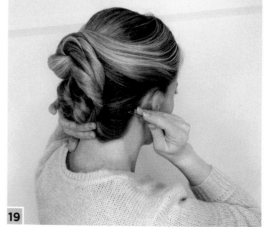

19

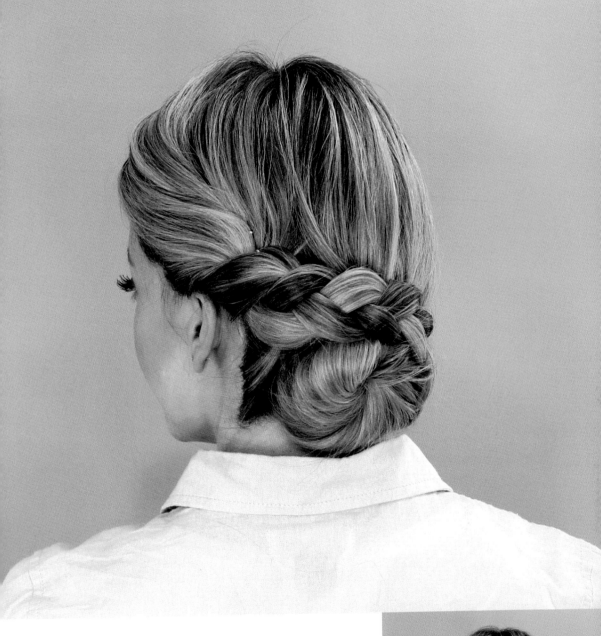

Braid-Wrapped Side Bun

Wrap your pretty bun with a gorgeous braid and jazz it up a notch. This hairstyle features a regular braid so there aren't any tricky techniques involved, and adding a braid to any style is a simple way to upgrade your look. Grab some pins and get ready to conquer the Braid-Wrapped Side Bun!

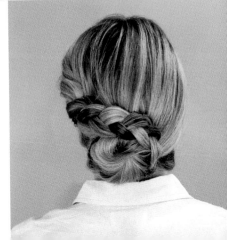

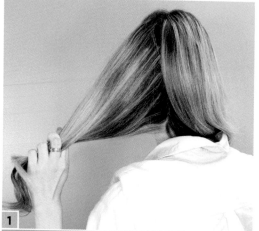

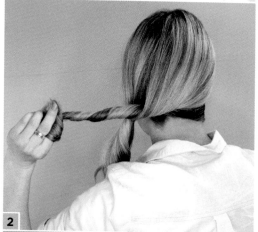

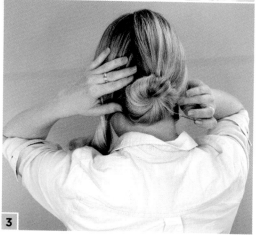

MATERIALS

» Wide-tooth comb
» 1 clear elastic band
» Maximum-hold hairspray
» 5–6 bobby pins

1. Comb through the hair to remove any tangles before dividing it into two sections, one larger than the other, from the crown down to the left side, at the nape of the neck. Use a clear elastic band to secure the left section while you work with the rest of the hair.

2. Take the right portion of hair and twist it all together downwards. For a sleek style, smooth the hair down with hairspray and a comb before twisting it.

3. Wrap the twist clockwise into a bun and secure the four "corners" with one bobby pin apiece. Use more if needed, but hide the pins by sliding them in towards the center of the bun.

4. Take out the left section of hair and create a braid by dividing the hair into three strands and crossing the side pieces over the middle.

5. Lay the braid over the top of the bun and wrap it around the bun, clockwise, pinning the end down with bobby pins. Liberally spray the style with hairspray to set it.

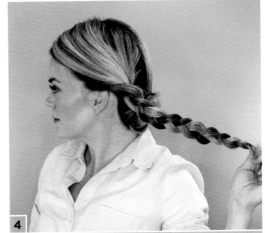

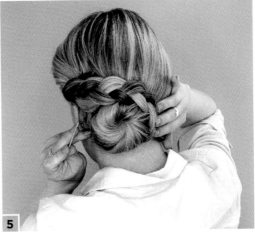

UPDO EXTRAS

Create extra volume by back-combing the hair at the crown before getting started. Smooth down the top layer to hide the teased portion. Also, when wrapping the hair for the bun create a smaller bun at first because it can always be made larger later on by gently pulling on the edges. It's also a good idea to tie off the braid with a hair elastic before wrapping it to ensure it doesn't come loose throughout the day; after creating the braid, gently pull on the edges to make it fuller.

CHAPTER 5

Knots, Twists, and Ponytails

Adding a knot or twist to any hairstyle can really help jazz up your look. Styles like the Knotted Updo, Twisted Mohawk, and Headband Hair Tuck—all found in this chapter—are modern and trendy ways to add detail and structure that will surely impress your family and friends. In addition, you'll also find some great new ways to amp up that ponytail to make it fun and flirty in no time. To ensure that your look—whether you're wearing a knot, twist, ponytail, or some combination of the three—is sleek and smooth, be sure to keep a little hairspray nearby for taming down frizz and flyaways.

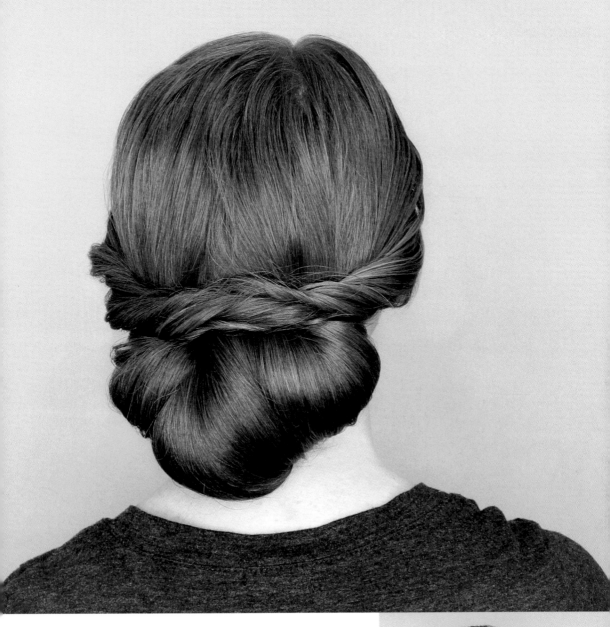

Twist Wrap Chignon

A gorgeous new updo that is perfect for that special occasion, school dance, or formal night out, this Twist Wrap Chignon features a chic low bun and two wrapped twists, which look complicated but are easy to create when you take a look at the quick steps. Top off this hairstyle with a beautiful crystal clip and you will be ready to hit the town.

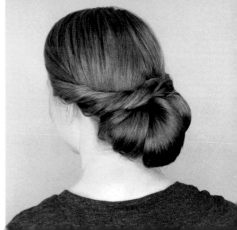

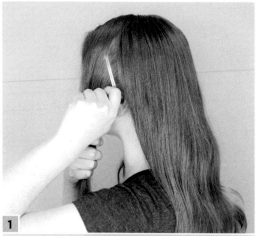

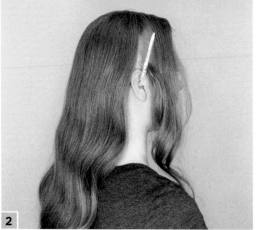

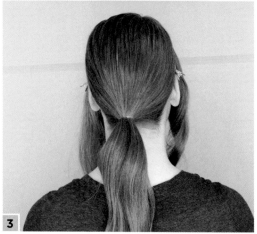

MATERIALS

» Wide-tooth comb
» 2 duck-bill clips
» Maximum-hold hairspray
» 2 clear elastic bands
» 10–12 bobby pins

1. Begin by creating a side part on the left side. Then, section off a portion of hair from the part down to the left ear. Clip off the front portion of hair with a duck-bill clip.

2. Repeat the previous step with the hair on the right side, clipping off the forward portion of hair with a duck-bill clip.

3. Comb through the back portion of hair, spray it with hairspray, and comb through it once more. Now tie the hair into a low ponytail with a clear elastic band.

4. Pull the ponytail slightly loose and create a gap in the hair directly above the elastic. Then loop the ponytail upwards, through the gap, into an upside-down topsy tail so the ponytail goes up and out of the gap.

5. Comb through the ponytail, mist it with hairspray, and comb through it once more to smooth down any flyaways. Tie a clear elastic over the end of the ponytail a few inches up from the bottom.

6. Lift up the top part of the ponytail and pin the hair against the head, just above the topsy tail.

7. Take the bottom part of the ponytail, at the elastic, and roll the hair up underneath itself to create the looped bun.

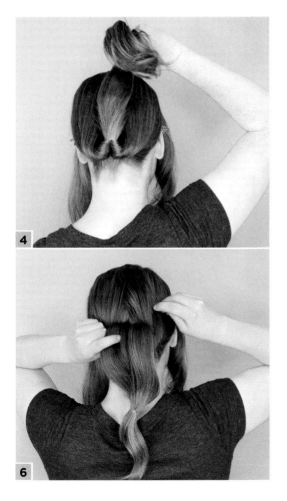

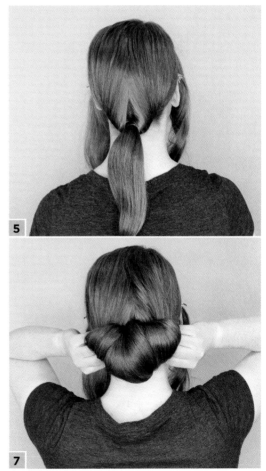

8. Pin down the bun, sliding the pins in horizontally so they are hidden under the bun.

9. Let down the hair that's clipped on the right side. Smooth it down by combing through it, misting it with hairspray, and combing through it again. Then twist the hair upwards and lay it across the top of the bun.

10. Wrap the twist around the left side of the bun, pinning it down, sliding the pin inwards under the bun.

11. Let down the hair that's clipped on the left side. Smooth it down by combing through it, misting it with hairspray, and combing through it again. Then twist the hair upwards and lay it across the top of the bun.

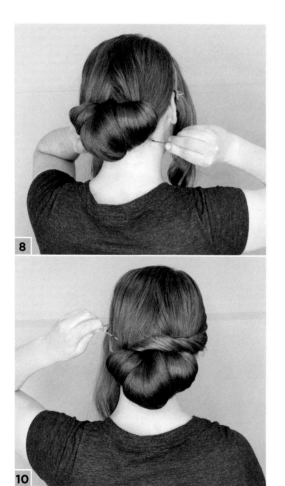

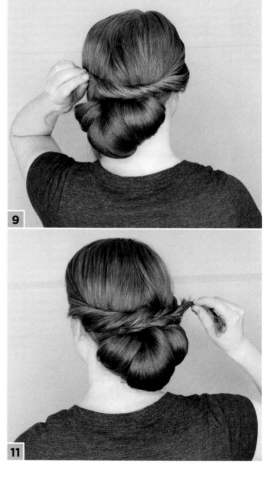

12. Wrap the twist around the right side of the bun. Pin down the end of the twist, hiding the pin under the bun. Liberally spray the style with hairspray to set it and ensure that it stays in place all day or evening.

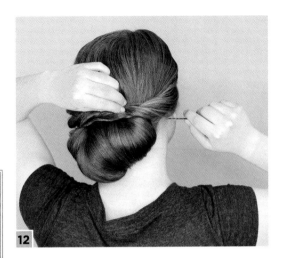

UPDO EXTRAS

After twisting the side sections, gently pull on the edges to create a softer, fuller twist before wrapping them over the bun.

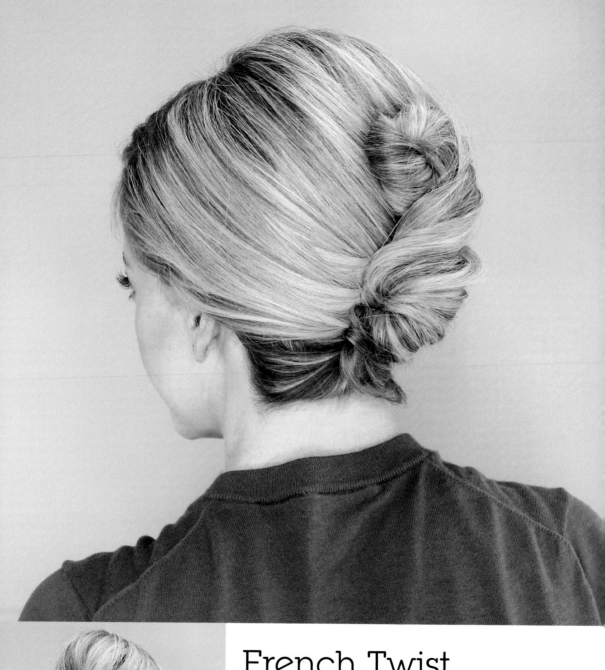

French Twist

A classic hairstyle that never goes out of style, the French Twist has made it through the ages and always looks glamorous whether it is worn to the office or to a formal occasion. You really can't go wrong with this one! Try it on second-day hair, when the hair already has some texture, and wrap it up in no time. This hairdo works great on any hair type, whether curly or straight, and looks flattering on just about everyone.

MATERIALS

» Teasing brush
» 6–8 bobby pins
» Medium-hold hairspray

1. Grab a teasing brush, separate off a small section of hair at the back of the crown, and gently back-comb the hair down. Repeat this with one more section, then gently smooth down the top layer of hair to hide the teased portion.

2. Combine all the hair together at the nape of the neck, brushing through it to remove any tangles. Then twist it all together, downwards.

3. Bring the twist upwards so it sits vertically against the head.

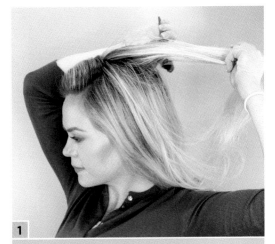

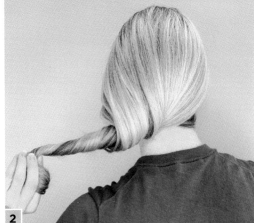

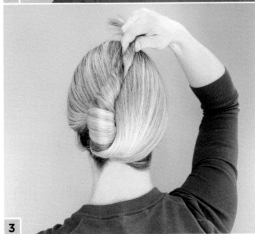

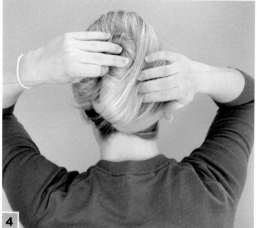

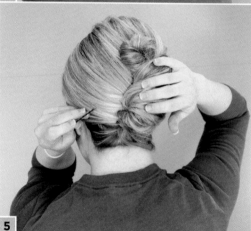

4. Keep a firm grip on the twist with your left hand, holding it against the head. Use your right hand to push the hair on the right side over the top of the twist, completely covering it if possible.

5. Place a firm hold on the hair with one hand and slide bobby pins into the fold with the other hand. The trick to hiding the pins here is to catch a tiny bit of hair with the open end of the bobby pin facing the left, then flip the bobby pin over itself, now facing towards the right side, and push it into the fold. Slide in as many pins as you need to until it feels secure. Then, spritz the style with hairspray and smooth a hand over the sides to ensure any stray hairs are laid flat.

UPDO EXTRAS

After twisting the hair, spray it with hairspray to ensure that it all stays together. If you have layers that stick out from the twist, simply pin them down after wrapping the hair.

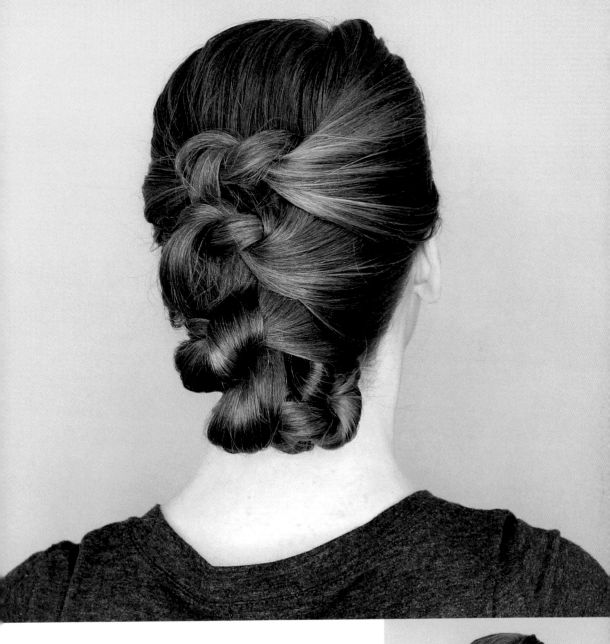

Knotted Updo

Try something new with this neat Knotted Updo! This hair-style is done by literally tying knots into the hair. Don't worry, they are easy to take out and, when tied one right after the next, create an intricate style that looks more complicated than it is. Give it a try and impress all your friends at your next party.

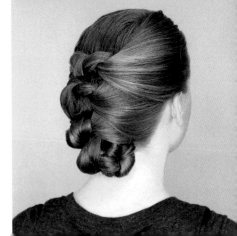

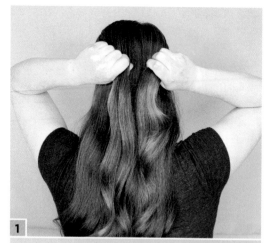

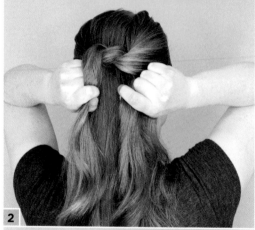

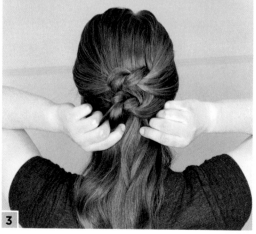

MATERIALS

» Wide-tooth comb
» 1 clear elastic band
» 4–6 bobby pins
» Maximum-hold hairspray

1. Comb through the hair to remove any snarls and tangles. Take sections of hair from both sides of the head, from the part down to the ears, and bring them towards the back of the head.

2. Create a knot by crossing the right strand over the left. Now that the strands have switched places, bring the right strand up and through the gap at the top, then back down. Carefully pull the two strands in the opposite direction to tighten the knot against the head.

3. Pick up a 1" section of hair on each side of the head, directly below the section from Step 1. Incorporate these sections into the two corresponding sections from the first knot so you still have one section on the right and one section on the left to work with. Create a second knot by crossing the right strand over the left, bring the right strand up and through the gap at the top, then back down again. Carefully pull the two strands in opposite directions to tighten the knot against the head.

4. Bring in the rest of the hair that is hanging down, so all the hair is incorporated into the sections being knotted. Tie a third knot, keeping it tight against the head.

5. Continue tying the hair into knots until you reach the end of the hair. Tie off the bottom with a clear elastic band.

6. Roll the hair under towards the nape of the neck. Pin the hair, securing it underneath, with bobby pins. Set the style by misting it with hairspray.

UPDO EXTRAS

Comb through the hair and spray with hairspray after tying each knot to keep the style sleek and smooth. To keep the knots from slipping, slide in a bobby pin or two to hold the style in place.

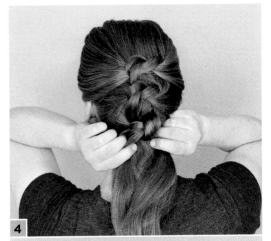

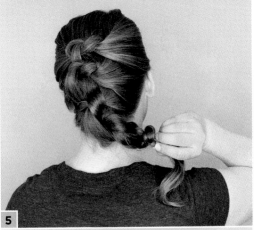

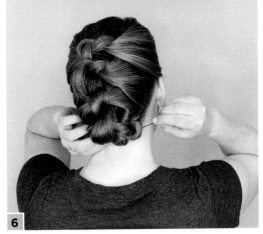

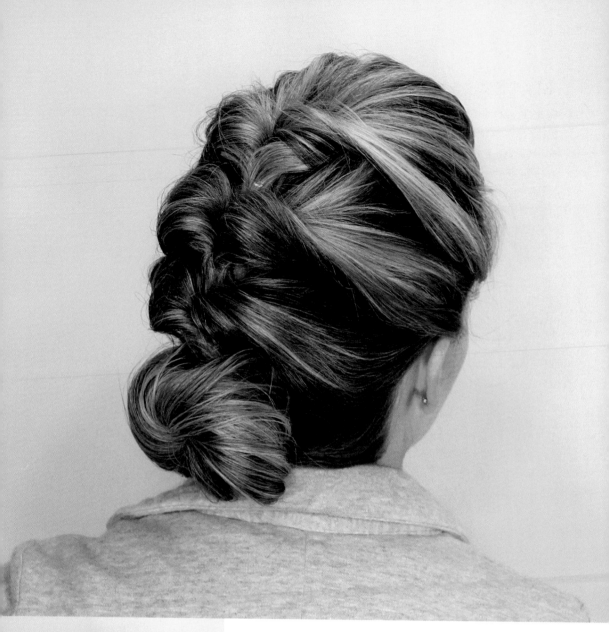

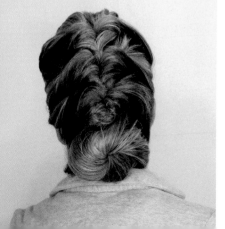

Twisted Topsy Tail Updo

What do you get when you combine three topsy tails and a chic bun? This Twisted Topsy Tail Updo! This hairstyle can take you from dull to dazzling, and it's easy to do but easier to learn. Let's get to it!

MATERIALS

» Wide-tooth comb
» 3 clear elastic bands
» 4–6 bobby pins
» Maximum-hold hairspray

1. Begin by picking up a section of hair, a few inches up from the ears and back to the top of the crown.

2. Tie off the section with a clear elastic band.

3. Create a gap above the clear elastic band for the topsy tail.

4. Flip the tail up and through the gap, pulling it back down tight.

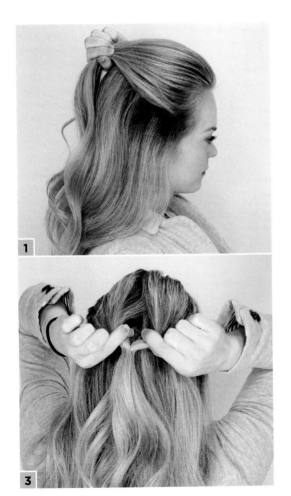

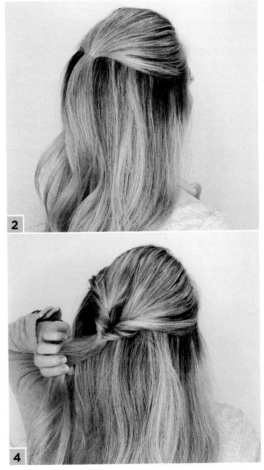

5. Gently pull on the edges of the topsy tail to close the space between each side.

6. Repeat the previous steps with two new sections of hair to create a second topsy tail directly below the first one.

7. Now create a third topsy tail a few inches above the nape of the neck.

8. Pick up the remaining hair and twist it all together.

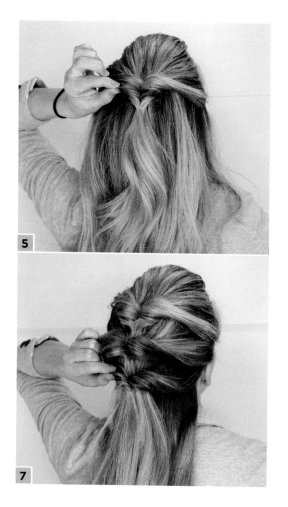

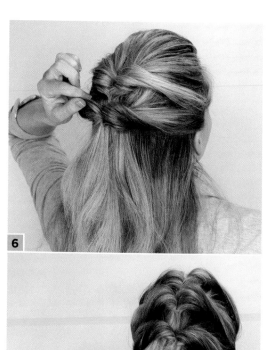

9. Wrap the twist around itself, forming a bun, and pin it against the head with bobby pins. Then set the style with hairspray and smooth down any flyaways.

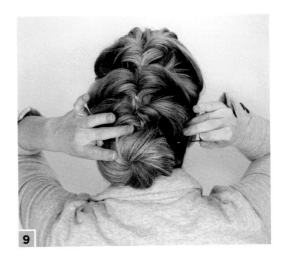

UPDO EXTRAS

Spray the hair with hairspray and comb through it before each topsy tail to ensure that the hair stays untangled and will look smooth and sleek in the end. Before creating the bun, spray the strands with hairspray and comb through them to remove any tangles.

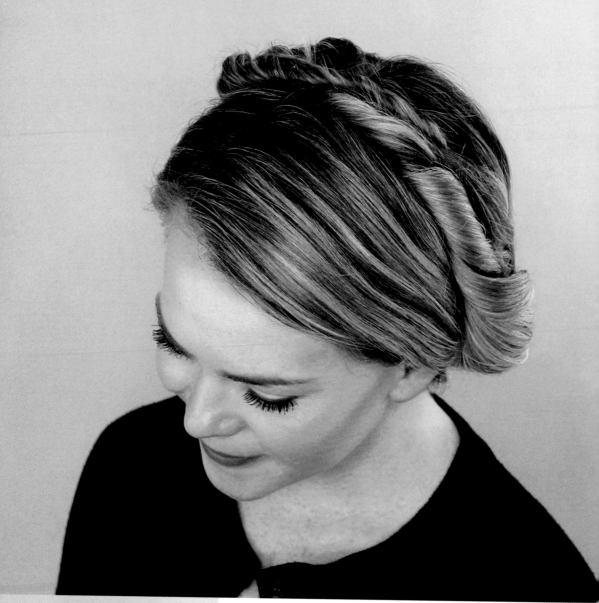

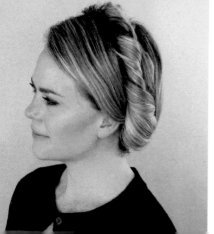

Twisted Headband

A modern version of the traditional Milkmaid Braids, this twisted 'do is ten times easier to do than that old favorite because there's not a braid in sight. Instead, this trendy Twisted Headband is created with two twisted sections, crossed over the head for a fun new spin. Let's get twisting!

MATERIALS

» Wide-tooth comb
» 2–5 bobby pins
» Maximum-hold hairspray

1. Comb through the hair before creating a part down the center of the back of the head, dividing the hair into two halves.

2. Take the left section and twist all the hair together upwards.

3. Lay the twist over the top of the head and pin it down with bobby pins. Be sure to pin down the very ends so they lie flat on top of the head.

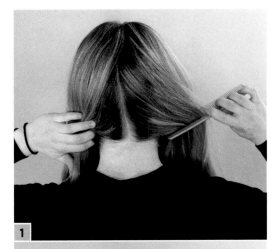

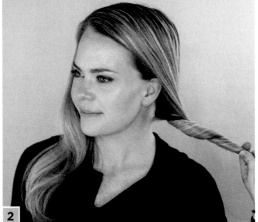

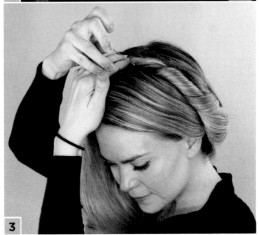

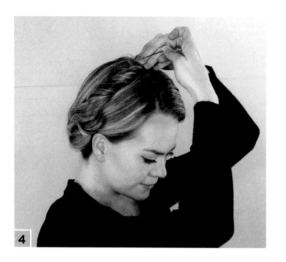

4

4. Repeat the previous two steps with the hair on the right side of the head. Lay the second twist over the end of the first twist, creating an "X" pattern. Then tuck the end of the second twist under the first one. Tucking the ends under the opposite twist will not only hide them but help make it look like one continuous twist. Then, mist the entire style with hairspray and gently smooth over any stray hairs.

UPDO EXTRAS

To ensure the style stays secure all day long, slide in pins along the entire twist; three or four should work perfectly.

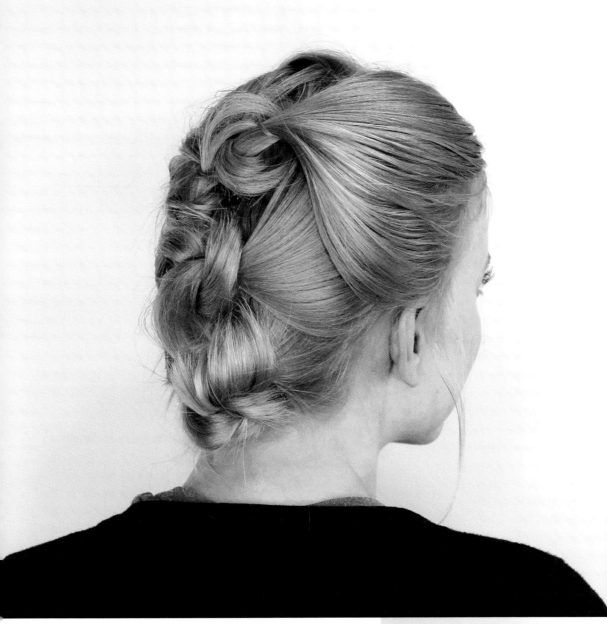

Twisted Updo

Change up your everyday style with this Twisted Updo. The hair is actually tied together in a bunch of little twisted knots to create this fun and unique style. Whether you're running to the store or out to dinner, this style is easy to do and even more fun to wear!

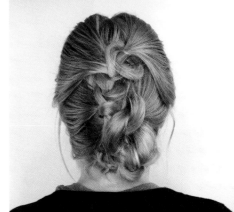

MATERIALS

» Wide-tooth comb
» 5–7 bobby pins
» Maximum-hold hairspray

1. Comb through the hair to remove any tangles. Pick up two small sections of hair from the front hairline and bring them towards the back of the head.

2. Tie the strands together by creating a half knot, looping one strand up and over the other.

3. Combine the two ends from this knot in your right hand and pick up a new section of hair on the left side of the head.

4. Create a second knot with the two sections you are holding and pull it tight against the head.

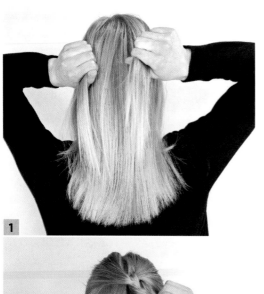

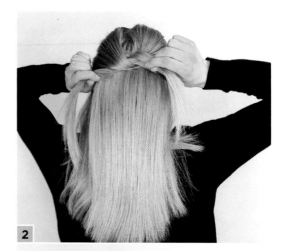

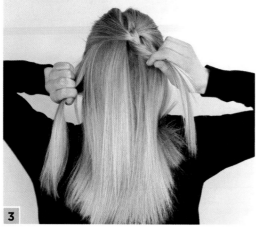

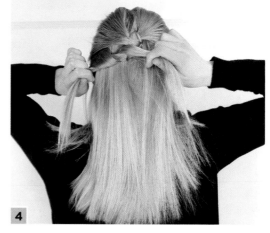

5. Repeat the previous steps—combining the two ends, picking up a new section of hair, and creating a third knot.

6. Pick up a 2" section of hair, behind the right ear. Then, using this new section and the section hanging down from the third knot, created in the previous step, tie a fourth knot.

7. Pick up the rest of the hair that is left hanging down. Use this as one section, along with the previously knotted section as the other, and create a final knot.

8. Roll the knot underneath and pin down the ends, hiding them underneath the bun created. Secure the knotted bun against the head with pins, then set the style with hairspray and run your fingers over each individual knot to lay down any stray hair or flyaways.

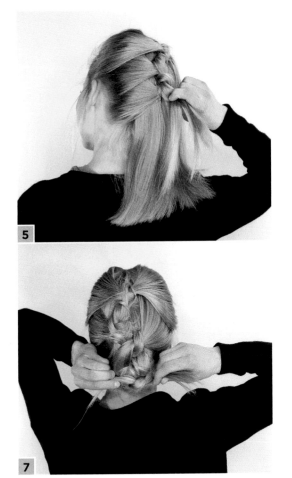

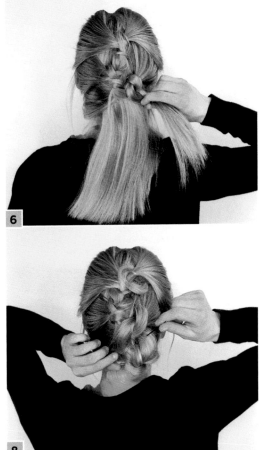

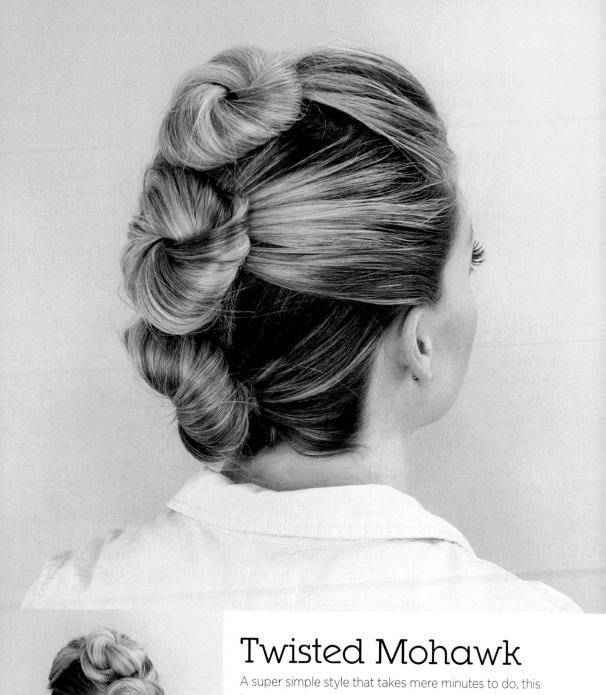

Twisted Mohawk

A super simple style that takes mere minutes to do, this Twisted Mohawk is perfect on second-day hair, especially if you have some leftover curls. Once you see how easy it is, you will wonder why you haven't tried it before!

MATERIALS

» Maximum-hold hairspray
» Wide-tooth comb
» 3 clear elastic bands
» 9–12 bobby pins

1. Separate off a section of hair, from the temples towards the top of the head. Spray the hair with hairspray and comb through it to ensure that it's smooth. Tie off this section with a clear elastic band.

2. Twist the tail and wrap it around itself into a bun, placing it directly over the clear elastic band. Pin it down with bobby pins, sliding them into the bun. Spray the bun with hairspray and smooth a hand over it to lay down any stray hairs.

3. Pick up a new section of hair at the top of the ears, bringing it towards the back of the head. Spray the hair with hairspray and comb through it to ensure that it's smooth. Tie off this section with a clear elastic band.

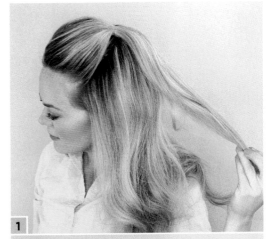

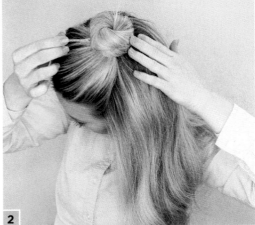

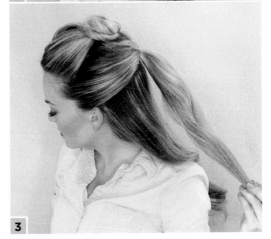

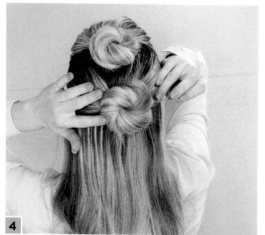

4. Twist the tail and wrap it around itself into a bun, placing it directly over the clear elastic band. Pin it down with bobby pins, sliding them into the bun. Spray the bun with hairspray and smooth a hand over it to lay down any stray hairs.

5. Sweep the remaining hair up into one more clear elastic band near the nape of the neck. Spray the tail with hairspray and comb through it to ensure that this last bun is smooth. Wrap the hair into a third bun, securing it with pins. Finish by misting the style with hairspray and flattening any stray hairs.

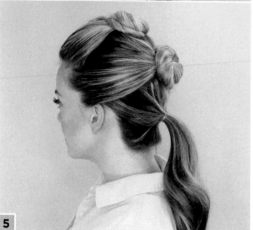

UPDO EXTRAS

Place each hair elastic close to the previous one to ensure there aren't any gaps between the buns. Once the buns have been created, gently pull on the edges of the buns to make them appear fuller.

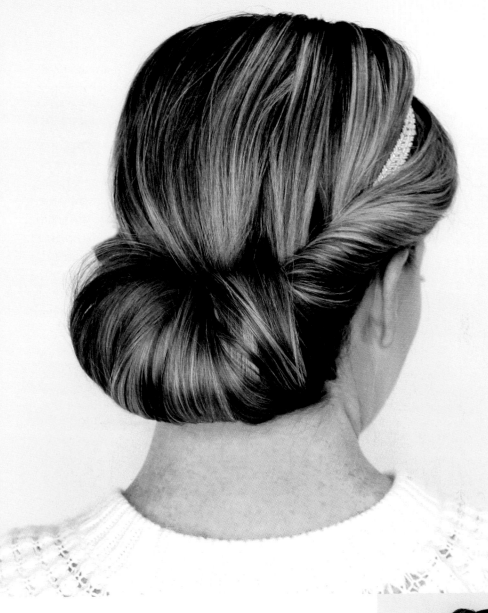

Headband Hair Tuck

A new and modern hairstyle that is so popular nowadays, this Headband Hair Tuck is super easy to do. It's the perfect hairstyle for any occasion and certainly for every day. Try it out—switch out your plain headband for a cute patterned one or something with sparkles for that special evening out. You and your friends will love this!

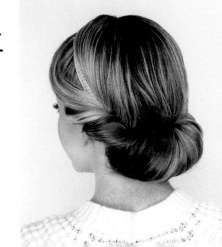

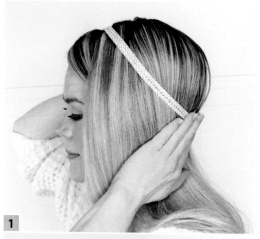

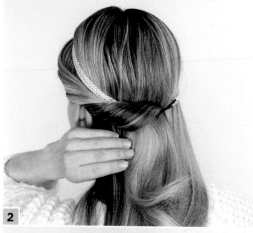

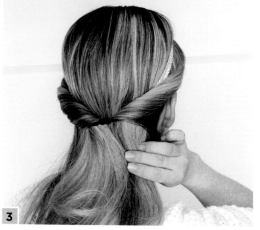

MATERIALS

» Wide-tooth comb
» Medium-hold hairspray
» Stretchy headband
» 1 clear elastic band

1. Comb through the hair, misting it with hairspray, to smooth down any flyaways. Place a stretchy headband over the head so it rests about 1" back from the hairline and 1" above the nape of the neck.

2. Pick up a section of hair from above the left temple and wrap it around the headband. Pull the hair down tight through the headband, then comb through it to remove any tangles.

3. Repeat the previous step with the hair on the right side, wrapping it around the headband and then combing through it.

4. Comb through the hair, spray it with hairspray, and comb through it once more. Wrap a clear elastic around the hair, about 4" up from the end.

5. Bring the tail up and tuck it into the headband. Keep tucking the hair so it creates a tight roll and all the hair is neatly tucked, then mist the style with hairspray to set it.

UPDO EXTRAS

To keep the headband from slipping off the head, slide in bobby pins at the base to ensure that it stays secure throughout the day. Also try misting the headband with hairspray before slipping it onto the head. This will help give it a bit of grip.

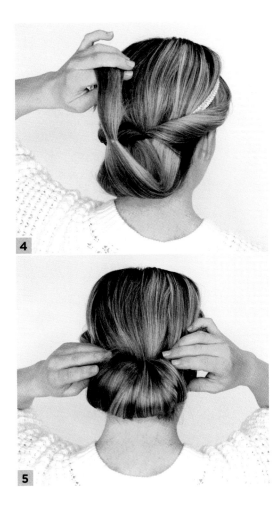

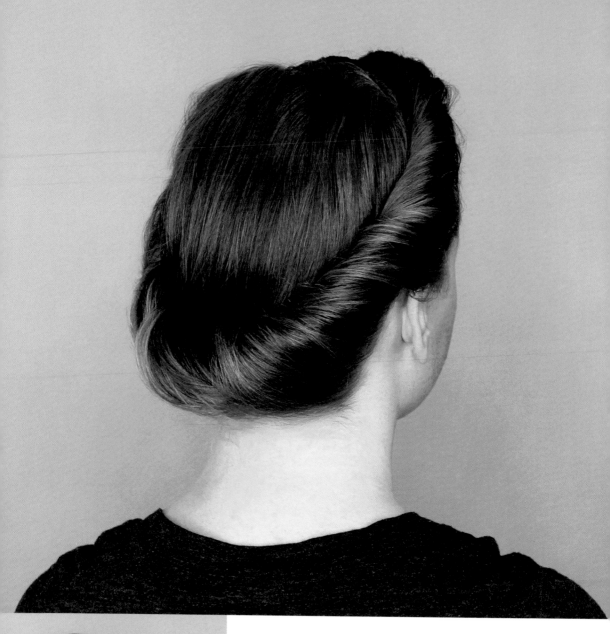

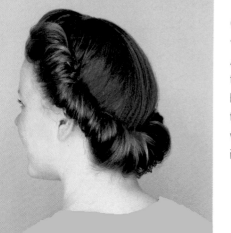

Spring Roll

All this style takes is a quick roll and you have a fun new way to wear your hair! If you love a pretty braid around the head but aren't keen on French braiding, then this Spring Roll is the perfect style for you. It only requires a bit of twisting and, with a few bobby pins, it stays in place and keeps you looking great throughout the day.

MATERIALS

» Wide-tooth comb
» Maximum-hold hairspray
» 3–5 bobby pins

1. Comb through the hair to remove any tangles. Mist the top of the head with hairspray and comb through it once more to smooth down loose hairs. Part the hair on the left side, then pick up a section of hair on the right side of the part and twist the hair towards the back of the head. Continue twisting the hair down towards the right ear and gradually bring in additional hair as you twist.

2. Continue twisting the hair down and around the nape of the neck before working the twist up the left side.

3. Bring the twist across the top of the head and tuck the ends underneath the beginning of the twist.

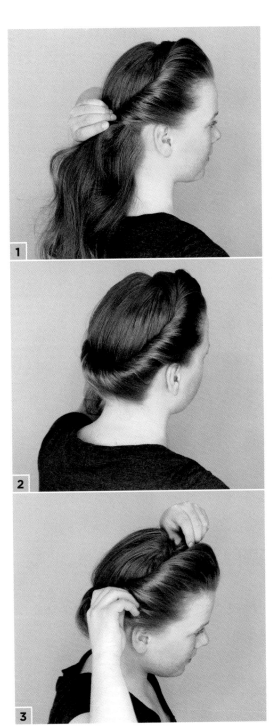

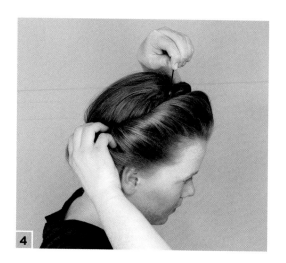

4

4. Pin down the end of the twist by sliding bobby pins under the roll. Then liberally spray the style with hairspray and smooth down any loose hairs.

UPDO EXTRAS

Comb through the hair before adding it into the twist. This will remove any tangles and ensure the final style is polished.

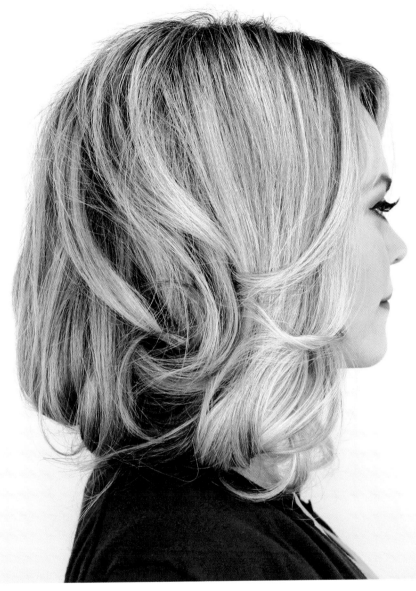

Faux Bob

Do you dream of short hair but don't have the guts to chop off your locks? Me too. That's where this Faux Bob comes in handy. The Faux Bob lets you fake a cute, short bob while keeping your long luscious strands at the same time!

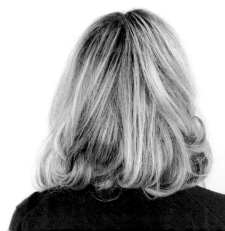

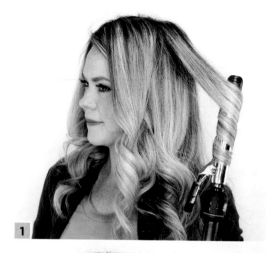

1

MATERIALS

» 1" curling iron
» 6–8 bobby pins
» Flexible-hold hairspray

1. Use a 1" curling iron to curl all the hair away from the face.

2. Separate out a 2" section of hair at the back of the head, slightly off-center towards the left side. Twist it upwards slightly to combine the section together so it's easy to wrap in the next step.

3. Roll the twist under and up towards the nape of the neck, creating a spiral-shaped mini bun.

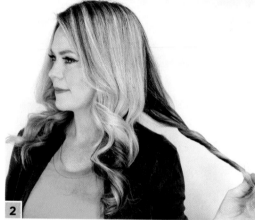

2

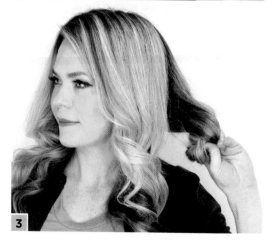

3

4. Tuck the mini bun underneath so it's against the head, at the nape of the neck. Pin the bun against the head using bobby pins. Make sure the pins are hidden underneath the hair.

5. Continue separating out sections of hair, rolling them under towards the nape of the neck and pinning them against the head.

6. To ensure each section is secure, criss-cross the bobby pins so they form an "X" underneath the hair. Then set the style with hairspray and run your fingers over the top of the hair to smooth down stray hairs.

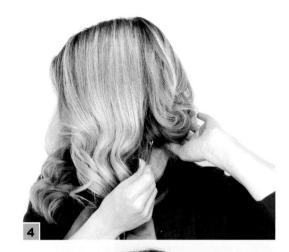

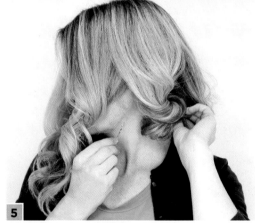

UPDO EXTRAS

To add a little extra volume to this style, back-comb the hair at the crown, then curl the hair in 1" sections to ensure that each strand is evenly curled.

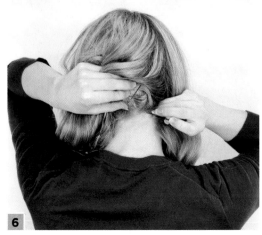

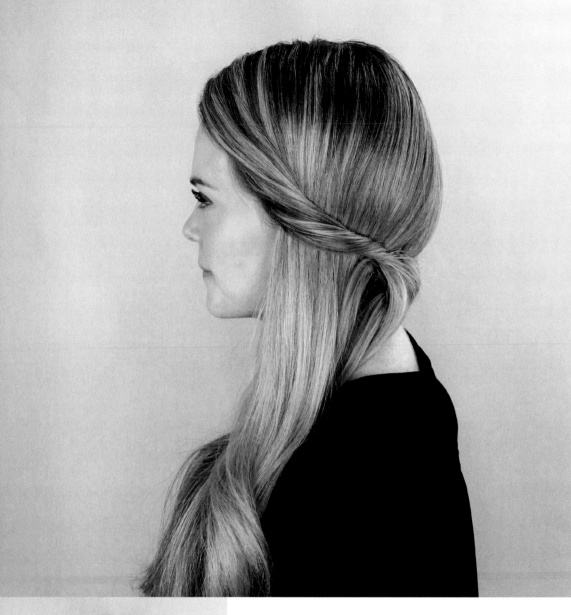

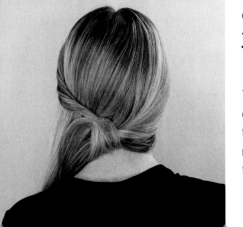

Side-Swept Wrapped Style

This Side-Swept Wrapped Style is a great way to wear your hair down but still dress it up a bit. With a few twists here and there this style is a cross between a ponytail and half updo, which makes this super easy and quick to do. Throw some curls into the ends of your hair and you'll be ready to hit the town!

MATERIALS

» Wide-tooth comb
» 4–6 bobby pins
» Medium-hold hairspray

1. Comb all the hair over the left shoulder. Then create a twist starting behind the right ear and working towards the left, stopping at the nape of the neck, behind the left ear.

2. Slide a pin vertically into the twist and push it towards the right ear so it rests horizontally along the head. This will help the twist stay in place more securely. Add in two or three more pins if the twist isn't tight enough.

3. Pick up a small section of hair, along the hairline on the left side of the head, from the part down to the left ear. Twist the entire section upwards, towards the back of the head.

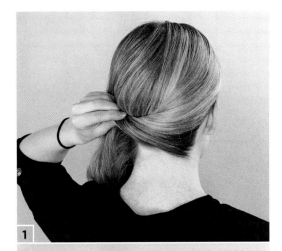

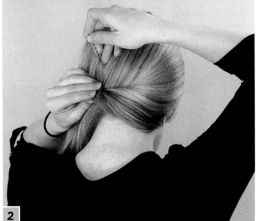

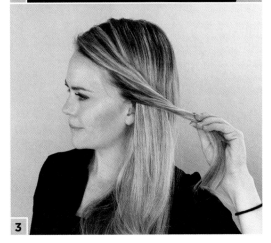

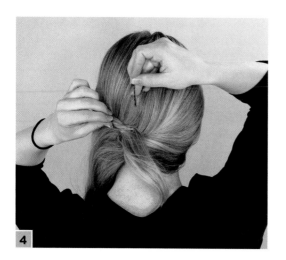

4

4. Pin this section so it meets at the first twisted piece. Then spritz the style with hairspray and smooth the hair over the shoulder again.

UPDO EXTRAS

Use a curling iron with a larger barrel, 1½", to create a wave in the hair, or create a tight curl with a smaller 1" curling iron before beginning the hairstyle. You can also back-comb the hair at the crown to add a little volume before beginning the style.

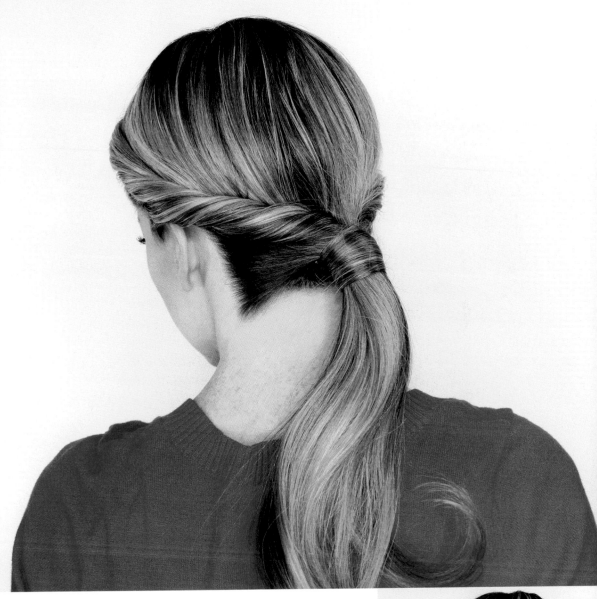

Twisted Low Ponytail

Are you bored with that everyday ponytail? Tired of throwing your hair into one whenever you don't know what else to do? Well, now you can dress it up with this sleek style! Two twists on each side of the head is quick and easy to do. Wrap it all together into a chic low ponytail and you have a great style for every day and every occasion.

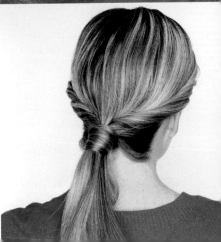

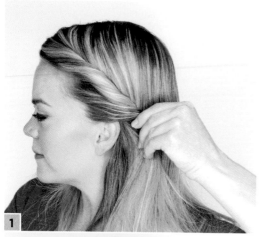

MATERIALS

» Wide-tooth comb
» Medium-hold hairspray
» 1 clear elastic band
» 3–4 bobby pins

1. Comb through the hair to remove any tangles, then mist the crown with hairspray and smooth it down. Take a 1" section of hair at the hairline on the left side of the part and begin twisting it upwards. Gradually bring in small sections of hair from above the twist and along the hairline, twisting the section towards the top of the left ear.

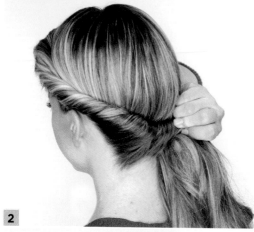

2. Continue twisting the hair around the back of the head towards the nape of the neck. Slide a few pins into the twist to hold it in place against the head.

3. Repeat the previous steps on the other side of the head, twisting the hair upwards to the nape of the neck.

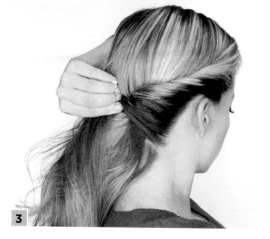

4. Secure the two twists together into a low ponytail at the nape of the neck with a clear elastic band.

5. Comb through the ponytail to remove any tangles. Then take a small section of hair from underneath the ponytail and wrap it around the clear elastic band to hide it.

6. Pin down the end of the wrapped hair, sliding in the pin towards the middle of the ponytail to hide it. Then set the style with a blast of hairspray and use your hand to smooth down any loose hairs.

UPDO EXTRAS

Once the style is set, curl the ends of the ponytail with a curling iron for a more polished look.

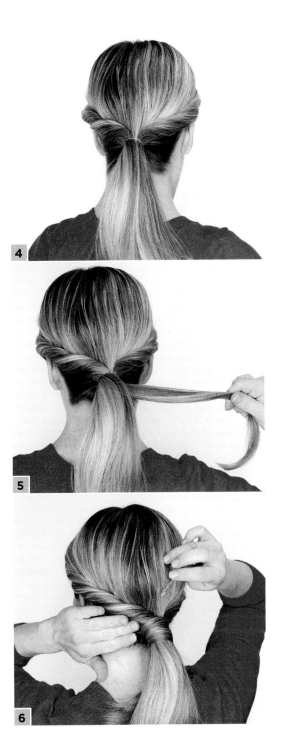

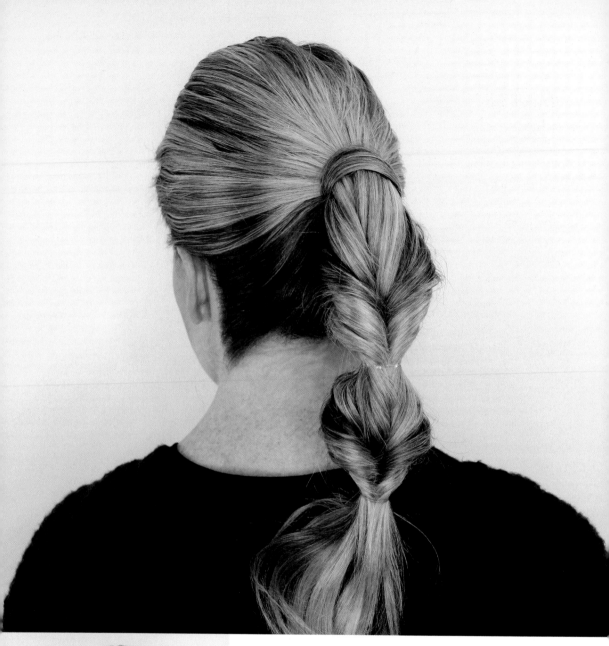

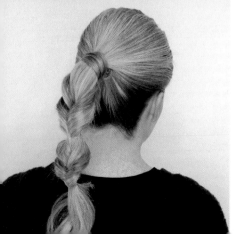

Topsy Tail Ponytail

If you're looking for a new way to wear an old classic, give this Topsy Tail Ponytail a try! All you need are a few elastic bands and a couple of flips and you have a jazzy new every-day ponytail. This style may look tricky but it is actually really easy to do. Once you get the topsy tail down, this sleek style will have all your friends staring.

MATERIALS

» Wide-tooth comb
» Medium-hold hairspray
» 3 clear elastic bands
» 1–2 bobby pins

1. For a sleek style, comb through the hair, spray it with hairspray, and then comb through it again. Now comb all the hair back into a ponytail, slightly above the ears, and tie it off with a clear elastic band.

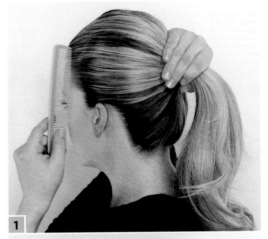

2. Take a small section of hair from underneath the ponytail and wrap it around the clear elastic band.

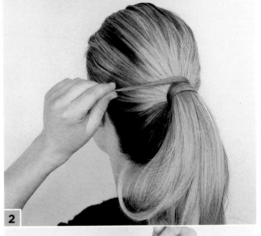

3. Slide a bobby pin over the tail of the wrapped piece and slip it under the ponytail to secure it.

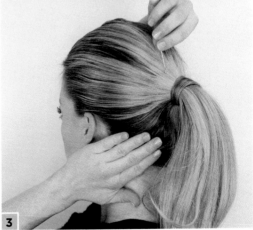

4. Wrap a clear elastic band around the ponytail, 2–3" down from the base.

5. Create a gap in the hair just above the elastic.

6. Flip the ponytail through the gap and pull it down tight to create the first topsy tail.

7. Wrap another clear elastic around the ponytail, 2–3" down from the previous one.

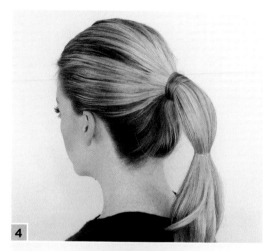

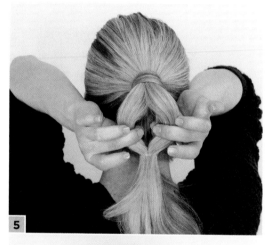

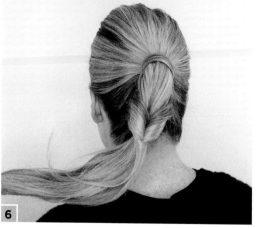

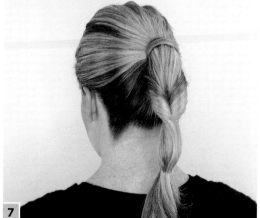

8. Create a second topsy tail by creating a gap above the elastic and flipping the tail through it before pulling it down tight.

9. Loosen the topsy tails by gently pulling on the edges to add volume and make them appear fuller. Then mist the style with hairspray to set it.

UPDO EXTRAS

Curl the ends of the hair with a curling iron to create a polished finish.

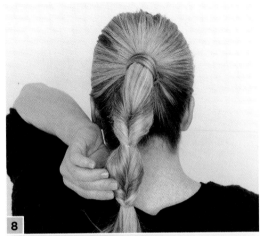

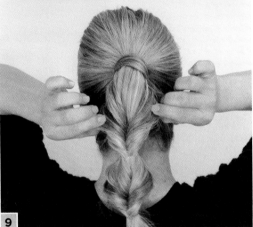

Index

Note: Page numbers in *italics* indicate specific hairstyles.

About the Author

MELISSA COOK is the creator of the blog *Missy Sue*. She is a happily married mother of two—to her son Cohen and Yorkshire terrier Gucci. She started blogging as a way to express her creativity and, hopefully, to one day be her own boss. Melissa has been sharing her passion for beauty and fashion for the past four years. She currently resides in Utah,1 where she hopes to inspire her readers to love their hair, develop useful makeup techniques, and celebrate everyday beauty. For video tutorials on more styles, check out her YouTube channel, *www.youtube.com/msncook11*, and visit her at *www.missysue.com*.